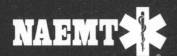
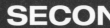

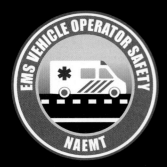

# EMS Vehicle Operator Safety

**Bob Elling, MPA, Paramedic (retired)**
Editor/Author

**Robert Raheb, AS, Paramedic (retired)**
Editor/Author

**National Association of Emergency Medical Technicians**
Reviewer/Endorser

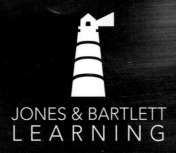

JONES & BARTLETT
LEARNING

*World Headquarters*
Jones & Bartlett Learning
25 Mall Road
Burlington, MA 01803
978-443-5000
info@jblearning.com
www.jblearning.com
www.psglearning.com

Jones & Bartlett Learning books and products are available through most bookstores and online booksellers. To contact the Jones & Bartlett Learning Public Safety Group directly, call 800-832-0034, fax 978-443-8000, or visit our website, www.psglearning.com.

Substantial discounts on bulk quantities of Jones & Bartlett Learning publications are available to corporations, professional associations, and other qualified organizations. For details and specific discount information, contact the special sales department at Jones & Bartlett Learning via the above contact information or send an email to specialsales@jblearning.com.

28827-8

**Production Credits**
Vice President, Product Management: Marisa R. Urbano
Vice President, Content Strategy and Implementation: Christine Emerton
Director, Product Management: Laura Carney
Director, Content Management: Donna Gridley
Manager, Content Strategy: Tiffany Sliter
Content Strategist: Ashley Procum
Content Coordinator: Michaela MacQuarrie
Development Editor: Heather Ehlers
Director, Project Management and Content Services: Karen Scott
Manager, Program Management: Kristen Rogers
Manager, Project Management: Jackie Reynen
Project Manager: Madelene Nieman
Senior Digital Project Specialist: Angela Dooley
Director, Marketing: Andrea DeFronzo

Marketing Manager: Elaine Riordan
Vice President, International Sales, Public Safety Group: Matthew Maniscalco
Director, Sales, Public Safety Group: Brian Hendrickson
Content Services Manager: Colleen Lamy
Senior Director of Supply Chain: Ed Schneider
Procurement Manager: Wendy Kilborn
Manufacturing Buyer: Bob Valentine
Composition: S4Carlisle Publishing Services
Cover & Text Design: Scott Moden
Senior Media Development Editor: Troy Liston
Rights & Permissions Manager: John Rusk
Rights Specialist: Liz Kincaid
Cover Image (Title Page): © Marco_Piunti/E+/Getty Images
Printing and Binding: Sheridan Kentucky

**Library of Congress Cataloging-in-Publication Data**
Names: Elling, Bob, author. | Raheb, Rob, author.
Title: EMS vehicle operator safety / Bob Elling, Robert Raheb.
Other titles: Emergency medical services vehicle operator safety
Description: Second edition. | Burlington, MA : Jones & Bartlett Learning, [2024] | Includes bibliographical references and index.
Identifiers: LCCN 2023035571 | ISBN 9781284291780 (paperback)
Subjects: MESH: Ambulances | Accidents, Traffic--prevention & control | Automobile Driving | Emergency Responders | Safety | United States
Classification: LCC RA995.5.A1 | NLM WX 216 | DDC 362.18/8--dc23/eng/20231030
LC record available at https://lccn.loc.gov/2023035571

6048

Printed in the United States of America
28 27 26 25 24    10 9 8 7 6 5 4 3 2 1

# Brief Contents

# Contents

# Acknowledgments

## Contributors

### EVOS Project Steering Committee

The following individuals were instrumental in creating the initial project proposal and shaping the scope of the EVOS first edition. We would like to thank them for their insight, experience, and contributions.

**Bob Elling, MPA, Paramedic (retired)**
Career Paramedic, Educator, Author, and EMS Advocate
Hernando, Florida

**Robert Raheb, AS, EMT-P**
Lieutenant Paramedic/Certified Instructor Coordinator, FDNY EMS (retired)
Career Paramedic, Educator, Author, and Speaker
New York, New York
Simulation Training Specialist, FAAC, Inc.
Miller Place, New York

**Anthony J. Deaven, EMT-P/ Firefighter**
Assistant Chief, Fire Aid and Safety Patrol
Lebanon, Pennsylvania

**Robert J. Faugh, EMT/Firefighter**
Rush Fire Department
Monroe County, New York

**David M. Reeves, MEd**
Fire Academy Director, Guilford Technical Community College
Jamestown, North Carolina
Captain, City Fire Department
Siler City, North Carolina

### NAEMT 2024 Board of Directors

Susan Bailey, President
Chris Way, President-elect
Troy Tuke, Secretary
Rob Luckritz, Treasurer
Bruce Evans, Immediate Past President
Rommie Duckworth, Director, Region I
Melissa McNally, Director, Region II
Shannon Watson, Director, Region III
Tim Dienst, Director, Region IV
Matt Zavadsky, At-Large Director
Douglas F. Kupas, MD, EMT-P, FAEMS, FACEP, Medical Director

### Second Edition Reviewers

**Debra L. Bell, MS, CCEMTP, EMT-T, NJ-CEM**
Atlantic Cape Community College – Paramedic Sciences
Atlantic City, New Jersey

**Trent R. Brass, MPH, RRT, EMT-P**
Rockford Fire Department
Rockford, Illinois

**Bradley Dean, MA, NRP**
Rowan County Emergency Services
Salisbury, North Carolina

**John Episcopo, NREMTP**
New York Presbyterian Hospital EMS
New York, New York

**Bruce S. Graham, Jr., BA, TP-C**
Virtua Health
Mount Laurel, New Jersey

**Bobbi Jo Henderson, EMTP**
Deputy Director of Education
Anderson County Emergency Medical Services
Clinton, Tennessee

**Greg P. Henington, Paramedic, FP-C**
Terlingua Fire & EMS
Brewster County, Texas

**Jordan Hronoski, Firefighter EMT, Instructor**
Hoyt Lakes Fire Department
Hoyt Lakes, Minnesota

**Richard Kaufman, MBA, NRP**
EMS West
Pittsburgh, Pennsylvania

**Justin Koper MS, FP-C, CSP, MTSP-C, DICO-C**
Director of Clinical Quality
EmergyCare
Erie, Pennsylvania
Adjunct Faculty, Bitonte College of Health and Human Professions
Youngstown State University
Youngstown, Ohio

**Daniel Lewis, MBA, NRP**
Indianapolis Emergency Medical Services
Indianapolis, Indiana

**Susan M. Macklin, MHA, Paramedic**
Central Carolina Community College
Sanford, North Carolina

**Nicholas McDaniels, MPA, NRP**
Johnson County Ambulance District Paramedic Program
Warrensburg, Missouri

**William G. McDonald, PhD, NRP, FACPE**
Staten Island Emergency Medical Training Center, Inc.
Staten Island, New York

**Jeremy Menzel, BS, NREMT-P**
Clayton County Fire and Emergency Services
Riverdale, Georgia

**Jonathan Oesterman, NRP, CCP-C**
Georgetown Scott County EMS
Georgetown, Kentucky

**Billy Petite, MEd**
Henry County Fire Rescue
McDonough, Georgia

**Lori Reeves, BA, PM**
Indian Hills Community College
Ottumwa, Iowa

**Mark Riley, NREMT-P, IC**
Tennessee CPR & EMS Education
Crossville, Tennessee

**Ronnie Swann, NREMT-P, FP-C**
UCHealth Lifeline
Denver, Colorado

**Jeri (Smith) Wheatley, Paramedic**
Division Chief of EMS
Arkansas City Fire-EMS Department
Arkansas City, Kansas

**Jeffrey A. White, MS, CHSP, MTSP-C, FP-C**
Director of Safety
HealthNet Aeromedical Services
Charleston, West Virginia

**Lt. David Wiklanski, MA, EMT(I)**
New Brunswick Fire Department
New Brunswick, New Jersey

## First Edition Reviewers

**Daniel Armstrong, DPT, MS, EMT**
Queensborough Community College
Bayside, New York

**Mark Baisley, MA, NRP**
Gold Cross Ambulance
Rochester, Minnesota

**Bruce Barry, RN, BSN, CEN, CPEN, NRP**
Peak Paramedicine, LLC
Wilmington, New York

**Debra L. Bell, MS, NRP**
AtlantiCare Regional Medical Center EMS and Inspira Health
Network EMS
Richland, New Jersey

**Trent R. Brass, MPH-EH, EMT-P, RRT**
SwedishAmerican Health System
Rockford, Illinois

**Charlene Cobb, NRP**

**Peter Dworsky, MPH, NRP, CBRM**

**Dan Evans, EMT, CIC, MA, MS**

**Scott A. Gano, BS, NRP, FP-C, CCEMTP**
Columbus State Community College
Columbus, Ohio

**Rob Garrett, MS, ASP, NRP**

**Greg P. Henington, NRP, LP**
Chief
Terlingua Fire & EMS, Inc.
Terlingua, Texas

**Paul Hinchey, MD**

**Ed Hollowell, RN, CFRN, CEN, NRP, CCP-C, FF**
Regional Fire & Rescue
Avondale, Arizona

**Scott A. Jaeggi, BA, EMT-P**
Instructor
Rio Hondo College Fire Academy
Santa Fe Springs, California

**K. C. Jones, NRP, NCEE**
Associate Professor
North Arkansas College
Harrison, Arkansas

**Rich Kaufman, MBA, NRP**
EMS Institute
Pittsburgh, Pennsylvania

**Sgt. Charles Kean, MA, EMT-P**
Springfield Police Department Emergency Response Team
Lincoln Land Community College
Springfield, Illinois

**Melodie J. Kolmetz, MPAS, PA-C, EMT-P**
Monroe Community College
Rochester, New York

**Daniel W. Lewis, MBA, NRP**
Indianapolis EMS
Indianapolis, Indiana

**Michael E. Lisa, BS**
NJ EMT/Instructor, Fire Officer (retired)
Trinitas Medical Center EMS Training
Elizabeth, New Jersey
Los Alamos Fire Department
Los Alamos, New Mexico

**Susan M. Macklin, BS, AAS, NC Paramedic**
Central Carolina Community College
Olivia, North Carolina

**Jeanette S. Mann, RN, BSN, NRP**
Director of Emergency Medical Services Program
Dabney S. Lancaster Community College
Clifton Forge, Virginia

**Donna McHenry, MS, NRP**
University of New Mexico
Albuquerque, New Mexico

**Taz Meyer, BS, EMT-P**

**Scott Miller**
EMS Program Director
San Jose City College
San Jose, California

**Keith Noble, MS, LP, NRP**
Commander
Austin-Travis County EMS
Austin, Texas

**Chris Ottolini, EMT-P, CPT**
Paramedic Supervisor, Coast Life Support District
Gualala, California
Adjunct Instructor, Santa Rosa Junior College Public Safety
Training Center
Windsor, California

**Allen O. Patterson, NRP, LP, CCP, EMSC**
Advance Coordinator
Lamar State College-Orange
Houston, Texas

**Paul Richardson, EMT-P**
Hancock County EMS
Carthage, Illinois

**Nicholas Russell, AAS, NRP, EMS-I, FI-3**
Edgewood Fire/EMS
Edgewood, Kentucky

**T. Troy Salazar, BS, OM; NRP; AZ, CO, NM Paramedic**
Southwest Colorado Community College
Durango, Colorado

**Jason Schiederer, MS, NRP**

**Jared C. Schoenfeld, CCEMTP, PNCCT, NRP**
Regional Transport Service
Mission Hospital
Asheville, North Carolina

**Bradley L. Spratt, MEd, LP, CSP**
Northwest Technical Solutions
Katy, Texas

**Robert Stakem, BS, CCEMTP, NCEE**
Harrisburg Area Community College
Harrisburg, Pennsylvania

**Daniel A. Svenson, BA, RN, NRP**
Portland Fire Department
Portland, Maine

**Michael Szczygiel, BS**

**Sara VanDusseldorp, NRP, CCEMTP, NCEE**
North Lake County EMS
Waukegan, Illinois

**Gary S. Walter, MS, NRP, EMSI**
International Rescue & Relief, Union College
Lincoln, Nebraska

**Roger G. Wootten, BS, NRP**
Northeast Alabama Community College
Rainsville, Alabama

## Photoshoot Acknowledgments

We would like to thank the following individuals and institutions for their collaboration on the photoshoots for the first and second editions of *EMS Vehicle Operator Safety*. Their assistance was greatly appreciated.

**Barry Bashkoff**
Cromwell Emergency Vehicles, Inc.
Clifton Park, New York

**Anthony M. Caliguire, NRP, CIC**
Paramedic Instructor Coordinator, HVCC Paramedic Program
Troy, New York
Lieutenant Paramedic, Scotia Fire Department
Scotia, New York

**Adam Henry**
Scotia Fire Department
Scotia, New York

**Danielle Matteo**
Bay Shore-Brightwaters Rescue Ambulance, Inc.
Bay Shore, New York

**Doug Ruso, EMT**
Albany, New York
Bay Shore-Brightwaters Rescue Ambulance, Inc.
Bay Shore, New York
Hudson Valley Community College
Troy, New York
Scotia Fire Department
Scotia, New York

# Dedication

Bob and Rob would like to dedicate this book to all the dedicated EVOs and EMS providers who have died in an emergency vehicle crash. Their passion to help others in their time of need should never be forgotten.

Bob would like to thank his mentor and lifelong friend Barry Bashkoff, who spent over five decades as an EMS provider, paramedic, EMS instructor, and ambulance salesman in upstate New York. His dedication to the public and EMS communities was second to none. RIP, we will take it from here…

# Preface

## EVOS Training

Thousands of EMS vehicle crashes occur each year, which suggests a clear training gap that needs to be filled. Dedicated to continually improving EMS education, the editors and contributors of *EMS Vehicle Operator Safety* have used their collective knowledge and breadth of experience both in the field and in the classroom to design a robust and engaging EMS vehicle operator training course. Developed in partnership with the National Association of Emergency Medical Technicians (NAEMT), EVOS is a national program with an open format that allows jurisdictions and agencies to incorporate local laws and regulations and SOPs, making it a course that is credible, flexible, and relevant to EMS providers of all levels of training.

## Why EVOS?

### Course Aims

EVOS focuses on what matters most—creating and maintaining a culture of safety. Its paramount goal is to reduce crashes, injuries, and fatalities involving EMS vehicles and providers. Built on the most current research, this evidence-based course underscores that both vehicle dynamics and human factors contribute to collisions, and that certain behaviors must be changed in order to promote a culture of safe driving. EVOS emphasizes increasing the emergency vehicle operator's awareness and understanding of vehicle safety, and the critical importance of understanding local laws and SOPs. It challenges EMS providers to think critically by analyzing real-life scenarios and typical crashes, highlighting the specific hazards that lead to collisions and offering practical strategies to avoid them.

### Course Education Philosophy

The EVOS course philosophy is rooted in the belief that analyzing actual crashes offers invaluable lessons that can be applied to future vehicle operator training and behavior. It is essential to take the time to share best practices and the hard lessons learned from past errors so that others will not repeat them.

Vehicle collisions are *not* accidents. In fact, the National Safety Council refers to them as *preventable crashes*. EVOS firmly refrains from using the term *motor vehicle accident* because conscious choices and behaviors lead to collisions; they do not simply happen.

## Key Themes and Significant Research

The revision of the *EVOS* to create this *EVOS Second Edition* has focused on the following key themes that are addressed in multiple chapters of the book:

- The lights and siren paradigm is shifting.
- The scene is never safe: traffic incident management is essential, not just a "move-over law" or wearing a visible vest!
- Forget the Golden Hour, consider a maximum of 10 minutes on scene instead. You can't save time driving faster.
- Every EVO needs training by qualified FTOs.
- Work-related fatigue affects greater than half of EMS personnel. Quality sleep is essential to avoid errors!

The following important documents have helped to move the ball down the field of EVO training significantly and have been incorporated into this *EVOS Second Edition* in the appropriate chapters.

- Joint Statement on Lights and Siren Vehicle Operations on Emergency Medical Services (EMS) Responses (February 14, 2022).
- U.S.F.A. Emergency Vehicle Safety Initiative, FA-336/February 2014.
- U.S.F.A. Traffic Incident Management Systems, FA-330/March 2012.
- U.S. DOT NHTSA Office of EMS, Lights and Siren Use by EMS: Above All Do No Harm, NHTSA Contract DTNH22-14-F-00579, May 2017.
- U.S. DOT NHTSA, Fatigue in EMS Systems, DOT HS 812 767, August 2019.
- U.S. DOT NHTSA, Characterizing Ambulance Driver Training in EMS Systems, NHTSA Contract DOT HS 812 862, December 2019.
- Department of Homeland Security, Science and Technology Directorate, First Responders Group, Ambulance Driver Best Practices, Contract GS-10-F-0181J, August 2013.
- U.S.F.A. and F.E.M.A. EMS Safety Practices, FA-359/April 2022.
- National EMS Safety Council, Guide to Developing an EMS Agency Safety Program, 2017.

# Enhancing EMS Vehicle Operator Training

EVOS was designed and developed by a team of seasoned field practitioners and educators with a wealth of unique experience in EMS safety and vehicle operator training.

- Bob Elling has dedicated much of his career to attempting to quantify the ambulance crash problem and remediate it through policy and education changes. As a training coordinator with New York State EMS, he helped develop seat belt use policies and piloted a New York State–sponsored Emergency Vehicle Operator Course (EVOC) instructor course. He also published one of the first articles in the *Journal of Emergency Medical Services (JEMS)* on the topic of ambulance crashes and developed the Ambulance Accident Prevention Seminar, which was rolled out as a continuing education workshop and taught to over 20,000 EMTs. Throughout his five decades in EMS he has consulted on the development of numerous EVO educational videos, articles, and educational programs.
- Rob Raheb observed early in his 32-year EMS career that there were no standard criteria for driving emergency vehicles. When he became the lieutenant in charge of the New York City Fire Department Bureau of EMS (FDNY EMS) Emergency Vehicle Operator Course years later, he sought to enhance it by researching and studying the science and art of driving and becoming both an accident investigator and a New York State–certified EVOC instructor. He later developed a driving simulator program and, after conducting an 8-year study to explore its effectiveness, demonstrated that by providing participants with opportunities to build their judgment and decision-making skills, simulation training could offer immense value. Rob has written numerous articles and has spoken at state and national conferences about driver training and the negative effects of collisions on the individual and the community. Today Rob travels around the country teaching emergency vehicle operator training and promoting simulation training.
- EVOS was developed in partnership with the NAEMT as an initiative to expand the culture of EMS safety, as initially portrayed in the organization's EMS Safety course (currently in its third edition), into a program that addresses the EVO's specific needs. The NAEMT's EMS Safety Committee played a critical role by reviewing the EVOS course materials to ensure their alignment with current guidelines, techniques, and best practices of the EMS Safety curriculum.

The editors and contributors of EVOS sincerely hope that you will find the course a valuable part of your EMS education.

# National Association of Emergency Medical Technicians

The National Association of Emergency Medical Technicians (NAEMT) was founded in 1975 to serve and represent the professional interests of EMS practitioners, including paramedics, emergency medical technicians, and emergency medical responders. NAEMT members work in all sectors of EMS, including government service agencies, fire departments, hospital-based ambulance services, private companies, industrial and special operations settings, and the military.

NAEMT serves its members by advocating on issues that impact their ability to provide quality patient care, providing high-quality education that improves the knowledge and skills of practitioners, and supporting EMS research and innovation.

One of NAEMT's principal activities is EMS continuing education. The mission of NAEMT continuing education programs is to improve patient care through high-quality, cost-effective, evidence-based education that strengthens and enhances the knowledge and skills of EMS practitioners.

NAEMT strives to provide the highest-quality continuing education programs. All NAEMT continuing education programs are developed by highly experienced EMS educators, clinicians, and medical directors. Course content incorporates the latest research, newest techniques, and innovative approaches in EMS learning. All NAEMT continuing education programs promote critical thinking as the foundation for providing quality care. This is based on the belief that EMS practitioners make the best decisions on behalf of their patients when given a sound foundation of evidence-based knowledge and key principles.

Once developed, continuing education programs are tested and refined to ensure that course materials are clear, accurate, and relevant to the needs of EMS practitioners. Finally, all continuing education programs are regularly updated no less than every 4 years to ensure that the content incorporates the most up-to-date research and practices.

NAEMT provides ongoing support to its instructors and the EMS training sites that hold its courses. Over 2,500 training centers, including colleges, EMS agencies, hospitals, and other medical training facilities located in the United States and more than 85 other countries, offer NAEMT continuing education programs. NAEMT headquarters staff work with the network of continuing education program volunteers from committee members; national, regional, and state coordinators; and affiliate faculty to provide administrative and educational support.

# CHAPTER 1

# Introduction to EMS Vehicle Operator Safety

## OBJECTIVES

**1.1** Outline the history of emergency vehicle operator training.

**1.2** Explain the need for an emergency medical services (EMS) vehicle operator course.

**1.3** Describe the profile of a "typical" ambulance crash.

**1.4** Explain the goals of the EMS Vehicle Operator Safety (EVOS) course.

**1.5** Discuss the changing views on the use of lights and siren (L&S).

**1.6** Describe the emergency vehicle operator selection process.

**1.7** Explain the value of analyzing cases of EMS vehicle crashes.

## SCENARIO

You pick up an extra midnight shift at your part-time medic job in Flushing, New York. Tomorrow is your day off at your full-time medic job in Manhattan, so you can go home and sleep in the morning. Since midnight, it has been quiet, and you are only on your second call. It is 3:00 AM and you and your partner, Pete, are transporting a 72-year-old woman to the hospital. She has a chief complaint of chest pain with a long cardiac history, so you have her resting in a semi-Fowler's position on your stretcher as you head to the emergency department (ED). You have already done an assessment and are following the STEMI protocol and have transmitted the 12-lead ECG to the ED. After administering care, you turn to some light conversation about her grandchildren to calm her down. Your partner is driving with his seatbelt on because your service's standard operating procedures (SOPs) require it, and you both know that it is good practice. You are seated on the crew bench, and the life-pack monitor is sitting on the bench next to you. Neither you nor the device is restrained, which is both legal and within the department policies.

As your partner proceeds through an intersection where he has the green light, another vehicle traveling at a high rate of speed runs the red light and the ambulance strikes the vehicle's left front quarter panel. In the moment when your partner sees the vehicle coming, he attempts to stop the ambulance and reaches for the brake as he screams, "Hold on!" Sitting in the patient compartment and in the middle of a conversation

*(continues)*

## SCENARIO (CONTINUED)

with the patient, you do not see any of the warning signs that the ambulance is about to collide with another vehicle. You and the patient are simply taken by surprise. The patient, who is restrained, is shaken up a bit but, fortunately, she does not leave the stretcher and the stretcher stays locked to the wall. You are not restrained and have nothing to grab to steady yourself, but even if there was a grab bar, with the amount of g-force exerted on the body, it would have been useless. You are thrown forward into the well between the driver's compartment and the patient compartment of this Type 3 ambulance. Everything happens so quickly. In an instant, you strike your head and are knocked unconscious; you do not see the airborne, 17.5-pound ECG monitor or feel it strike you in the lumbar spine. Fortunately, your partner is not rendered unconscious and responds quickly by bringing the vehicle to a stop before it hits a utility pole. His first act is to call for the police and two additional ambulances. Before he has a chance to get out and check on you, the other driver speeds away.

A short time later, as you regain consciousness, you hear a lot of commotion and see your friend Zack, a medic from Brooklyn. A crew is moving the elderly patient to another ambulance. Fortunately, she does not sustain any new injuries. You later learn that she was admitted to the critical care unit to be monitored on telemetry for the night. Although your ambulance is totaled, your partner experienced only a neck strain and minor glass cuts. After several hours, the police finally locate the drunk driver who crashed into your ambulance; he was driving with a suspended license. He had no injuries.

Your injuries include a broken thumb, a concussion, and two small fractures in your lumbar spine with no neurologic deficits. The back injury will result in a couple of weeks of light duty and a lifetime of intermittent back problems. All things considered, you feel lucky that this crash did not end your career. After some reflection, you realize that you learned a lesson you can share with other EMS practitioners for the rest of your career: Always be prepared for a collision by securing all equipment, and be sure you are *always* belted in during transport while in the patient compartment of the ambulance.

1. What were the preventable factors that led to this collision?
2. What factors were you unable to control that led to this collision?
3. Could the outcome have been the same had this scenario not involved a collision with another vehicle?

# History of Emergency Vehicle Operator Training

It has been well documented that emergency medical services (EMS) vehicle collisions cause significant injury, death, and property damage each year in the United States. Per data from the **National Highway Traffic Safety Administration (NHTSA)**, between 2010 and 2020, there were over 300 deaths resulting from ambulance-related crashes, with the majority of fatalities involving the occupants of nonemergency vehicles or pedestrians. Over the years, a number of training programs have been developed with the goal of better educating drivers of emergency vehicles in an effort to dramatically reduce the number of tragic accidents. The number one rule of medicine has always been, "First, do no harm." Yet, each year across the United States, patients, bystanders, family members, and EMS practitioners are killed or seriously injured during collisions involving ambulances. These collisions, injuries, and deaths do not discriminate based

on response variables: volunteer or paid staff, private or public agency, 911 response or interfacility transfer. Today, the Internet nearly guarantees that moments after a collision occurs the details will reach the news media, social media sites, and trade journal websites.

One of the first efforts to address the lack of standardized education for **emergency vehicle operators (EVOs)** was the U.S. Department of Transportation's (DOT's) development of the **Emergency Vehicle Operator Course (EVOC)**. The original 1978 course was general and designed to reduce the incidence of emergency vehicle collisions, so it included sections for police, fire, and EMS vehicles. The 1978 edition of EVOC was revised in 1995 to the *Emergency Vehicle Operator Course (Ambulance): National Standard Curriculum*. The revised curriculum addressed emergency vehicle operations as they relate to the operation of ambulances, and included both didactic and skills range components. There were some limitations and mixed opinions of EVOC. While some services did not believe they had the space or instructors to teach the program, other services have had success integrating some aspects of EVOC into their on-the-job training of new employees and retraining of those who were involved in a collision.

In 2011, the National EMS Advisory Council's (NEM-SAC) Final Advisory—Emergency Vehicle Operator Education, Training, and Safety, noted that ambulance operator training was not well characterized. NEMSAC made these recommendations to NHTSA:

1. NHTSA should assess the status of emergency vehicle operator training programs (courses) throughout the United States;
2. NHTSA should conduct studies to determine the efficacy and/or effectiveness of emergency vehicle operator training programs; and,
3. NHTSA should produce an action plan for improving emergency vehicle operator education and training for ground ambulances.

Given that the most recent NHTSA curriculum for EVOC was last updated and released in 1995 and there has been relatively limited research conducted specifically around ambulance operator training, NHTSA sponsored additional research to better understand the content and types of ambulance training across the country. Based on Internet surveys of local ambulance agencies, the study produced the following key findings:

- Eighty-seven percent of agencies that operated ground ambulances reported that their operators completed some form of emergency vehicle operator training, with 74% requiring some type of training.
- Roughly half of the agencies that reported using training courses said their programs were based on the NHTSA standard curriculum.
- Regarding content delivery, the majority of agencies incorporate a classroom component (>80%) and hands-on training (70%). Simulation and Internet-based courses were used by 5% and 15% of respondents, respectively.
- When ambulance operator training was used, only 20% of courses were longer than 20 hours, and 40% of courses were reported to be less then 10 hours of total training time.
- "Check rides," in which a senior staff member rides along to monitor operator fitness, were used in just over 55% of responding agencies. The most common evaluation components for these ridealongs were basic driving procedures, driving procedures under special circumstances (inclement weather, use of lights and siren, etc.), communication, vehicle staging, and vehicle readiness. Less than one-quarter of agencies using check rides evaluate fatigue management in their EVOs.
- Most agencies (~60%) require refresher training at least every 2 years, with almost 38% requiring

annual training. Over 16% reported offering no refresher training.
- Less than one-fifth of agencies require remedial training for all operators involved in a crash, with an additional 68% stating that remedial training is required on a case-by-case basis.

Given these high levels of variability in training, other programs were developed, such as the following:

- Since 1980, the Volunteer Firemen's Insurance Services (VFIS) has partnered with fire and EMS leaders to enable the continuing development of policy and program enhancements, specialized education, and consulting for management needs. The VFIS's program, called the **Emergency Vehicle Driving Training (EVDT)** program, was updated in 2016 to include new hands-on and knowledge-based training designed for both new and experienced drivers.
- In 1989, the **Ambulance Accident Prevention Seminar (AAPS)** was developed by New York State EMS Program staff under a Governor's Traffic Safety grant. This 1-day program was designed to improve attitudes toward and awareness of ambulance operator safety, presenting information on driving laws and common causes of ambulance crashes (but lacking a skills component). Nearly 25,000 practitioners were trained in the first few years; however, there appeared to be little success based on the number of collisions still occurring. Although the course was well received and awarded traffic safety awards, the program has not been updated.
- In the early 1990s, the National Safety Council released the first edition of **Coaching the Emergency Vehicle Operator (CEVO)**. It is currently in its Fourth Edition, and there are multiple specific courses offered: Fire Truck Driver Training, Ambulance Driver Training, and the Ambulance Driver Training Program for Maneuvering Skills. The courses teach defensive driving techniques to maneuver safely through traffic under severe time constraints and stress.
- Many services have developed their own versions of EVOC, based on standards from the Occupational Safety and Health Administration (OSHA), **National Fire Protection Association (NFPA)**, the 2009 *National EMS Education Standards,* and guidance from their respective states.
- In 2018, after years of development, the **EMS Vehicle Operator Safety (EVOS)** course was released. EVOS is endorsed by the National Association of Emergency Medical Technicians (NAEMT) as one of their series of very successful continuing education courses. The course addresses the vehicle operations and transport safety

knowledge gaps that lead to injury and death. Built on current research and featuring discussions of actual crashes and common driving scenarios—and the lessons that can be learned from them—it challenges EVOs to consider if they truly know how to arrive at a scene safely.

## Emergency Vehicle Operator Training Today

Although the term EVOC is widely used, there is a distinction that should be made. The NHTSA curriculum is referred to as EVOC, yet there are many courses that are "based" on the curriculum. In the 2019 NHTSA report, for the first time, a team of subject matter experts (SMEs) reviewed the 121 topics covered in the 1995 NHTSA EVOC curriculum. The topics were used as a "standard" to compare to other training programs, but it was also noted that the standard needed substantial updating in terms of both content and delivery approach. The SMEs felt that a controlled evaluation of the effectiveness of a state-of-the-art EVOC program designed specifically for ambulance operators would be beneficial. Developing such a program from scratch, however, would likely be expensive as it would involve the production of videos, computer-based training, and thorough vetting of on-road training approaches. A rigorous scientific study could also take years to conduct if ambulance crashes and patient outcome measures were to be collected. A more cost-efficient approach could involve evaluating an existing program that appears to represent the current state-of-the-art in-ambulance operation. EVOS was designed to help meet these needs.

## Safety in Emergency Vehicle Operations

### Estimates of the Depth and Breadth of the Problem

Hard numbers on emergency vehicle–related crashes can be difficult to come by, given the lack of a national consolidated database and publicly available information. Most statistics seem to be estimates or extrapolations based on limited data, though research from state-level databases can provide some idea of the extent of the issue, and historical data can be helpful in following trends over time.

In New York State (NYS), a series of deadly ambulance crashes led to a review of ambulance crash data (courtesy of the NYS Department of Motor Vehicles). Based on 28 years of NYS data, there were 9,599 ambulance collisions—an average of 343 per year. During this time, 78 persons were killed (an average of 3 per year) and 13,701 persons injured (an average of 489 per year). The profile of a "typical ambulance crash" includes clear weather, daylight hours, a right-angle lateral collision, a dry road surface, and an intersection that had a traffic control device.

These data reveal similar trends from a previous report, "Dispelling Myths on Ambulance Accidents," published in the *Journal of Emergency Medical Services* in July 1989, that covered an 18-year period in NYS. The data seem to repeat the same story, even after 10 more years of data have been added to the database.

In 2012, NHTSA released a 20-year analysis of ground ambulance crashes. The data were from a review of the 1992–2011 Fatality Analysis Reporting System (FARS) and National Automotive Sampling System (NASS) General Estimates System (GES). The national picture of the extent of the problem revealed the following summary:

- Average number of crashes involving a ground ambulance per year was estimated to be 4,500.
- Typical year included 33 fatalities, of which 4% were ambulance drivers, 21% were ambulance passengers, 63% were occupants of other vehicles, and 12% were nonoccupants.
- Typical year included 2,600 injured persons, of which 17% were ambulance drivers, 29% were ambulance passengers, and 54% were occupants of other vehicles.
- Almost 60% of both fatalities and injuries occurred during emergency use.

Even though the data are limited, it's clear that ambulance safety is still a major concern, almost 40 years later. However, without reliable crash information to compare, evaluating the usefulness of EVO training becomes almost impossible. In 2012, the Fourth Edition of the MMUCC (Model Minimum Uniform Crash Criteria) Guidelines was released to help states improve and standardize motor vehicle crash data. These guidelines suggest voluntary minimum criteria that police use for crash reports. For the first time in this edition, the ambulance attributes were expanded to include emergency/nonemergency transport, emergency operation/warning equipment in use/not in use, and ambulance seating/positioning. These changes, once incorporated into each state's reports, should help give a better picture of the problem of ambulance crashes.

There are also voluntary reporting websites where EVOs and practitioners can provide information on near-miss incidents (where a crash or injury was possible, but did not occur). These reports of crashes or close calls can then be used by other agencies as research or educational opportunities to avoid making similar mistakes. See Chapter 12 for more information on the various near-miss reporting systems.

# Human Behaviors

If you saw a paramedic starting an IV without wearing gloves, you would certainly notice the error and quickly point it out; however, you would not have felt the same concern in the 1970s. How was that mindset changed?

Ambulance design is constantly changing to improve safety, yet these vehicles are still dangerous for their occupants. The fact is, no matter how sound the design, construction, and mechanics of an ambulance, there will always be one uncontrollable component: the human being operating it. Emergency vehicles will be used in fundamentally unpredictable ways. It will be used to negotiate traffic (which is itself unpredictable) in an urgent manner while trying to obtain the right of way. It will be used to transport individuals, sometimes engaged in a desperate fight for survival, and their medical practitioners, who despite their skill and attention to safety protocols, will sometimes feel less inclined to worry about their own safety than the needs of their patients. EMS practitioners may disregard measures such as restraining themselves or their equipment in order to save seconds while working on patients; this can be a deadly choice. Just like their patients, EMS practitioners in the patient compartment of an ambulance are subject to all the laws of physics should a collision occur.

In addressing transport safety, the questions must not focus solely on vehicle dynamics but also must consider human dynamics. What human behaviors need to be changed for operators of the ambulance? What policies and procedures need to be developed to guide operator behavior? How can we instill a culture of safety in a profession with a history of taking chances to save lives?

An example of a pervasive safety issue that cannot be fixed by engineering is fatigue. The long hours and shift work inherent in EMS make staying well rested difficult under the best circumstances, but add in the stress of life-or-death responses and the mentality of pushing yourself beyond your limits for the sake of patient care, and it's no wonder fatigue is a concern. Although the EVO is ultimately responsible for ensuring they are well rested and fit for duty, the question then becomes, what else can be done to prevent the harm that can result? Increasing the punishment is one answer; in New Jersey, it's possible for a drowsy driver who accidentally kills someone to be charged with vehicular homicide (up to 10 years in prison and a fine of $100,000). Changes can also be made in the EMS system to prevent practitioners from overextending themselves; for example, administrators can limit the number of consecutive hours practitioners can work without a sleep break, and space can be made in the station specifically for resting. (See Chapter 2, *Making Safety a Priority*, for more information on fatigue and ways to limit its effects.)

However, even with the knowledge of the dangers, ambulance crashes are still far too common. Why is this human behavior not changing? This course, EMS Vehicle Operator Safety (EVOS), focuses on this important question and the following related questions:

- Do EMS agencies share best practices, such as policies, training programs, and public education, and learn from mistakes?
- Do services conduct motor vehicle record reviews on all ambulance operators?
- How much of a factor is the "hero mentality"— rushing to save seconds? Many EMS practitioners fall prey to the belief that arriving at the scene or the hospital 30 seconds earlier would make a difference in patient clinical outcome, although it rarely does.
- Are there best practices for use of lights and siren?
- Does better use of emergency medical dispatch protocols help reduce the number of emergency (lights and siren) responses? Jeff Clawson, MD, considered the "Father of Medical Priority Dispatch," thinks so.
- Is everyone really a good and safe driver? Is there a place in EMS for poor drivers?
- Are crashes an acceptable part of doing business?
- Is road rage and distracted driving increasing?

# Some Concerns and Some Progress

As research into ambulance design and responses grows, there will be better science to guide the construction of new units. Better designs coupled with changes in attitudes and behaviors should reduce ambulance crashes and associated morbidity and mortality. The **Centers for Disease Control and Prevention (CDC)** has begun to review the data on injuries to EMS workers. Recognizing that there is a problem is a good first step. Their research raises a number of critical questions; for example, it is no longer considered acceptable to drive the ambulance while intoxicated, but what about over-the-counter (OTC) medication use or driving while drowsy?

Another safety issue in EMS that has been undergoing change is the attitude toward racing to the call with **lights and siren (L&S)**. While research has consistently shown that the time savings from L&S response does not have an appreciable impact on patient outcomes, the 2022 EMS Trend Report indicated that the majority of EVOs believe that their use of L&S is appropriate; however, over three-quarters of respondents believe that use of L&S increases risk. While practitioners may be comfortable taking on the extra risks to themselves, it is critical to remember that patient safety is also at risk. To provide guidance to EMS agencies, 13 leading associations issued a joint statement on safely decreasing the use of L&S when appropriate (**Box 1-1**). In addition, the legal community, insurance companies, the CDC, and OSHA

**BOX 1-1  Taking a Stand for Safety: Joint Statement on Lights & Siren Vehicle Operations on Emergency Medical Services (EMS) Responses**

*Douglas F. Kupas, Matt Zavadsky, Brooke Burton, Shawn Baird, Jeff J. Clawson, Chip Decker, Peter Dworsky, Bruce Evans, Dave Finger, Jeffrey M. Goodloe, Brian LaCroix, Gary G. Ludwig, Michael McEvoy, David K. Tan, Kyle L. Thornton, Kevin Smith, Bryan R. Wilson*

**February 14, 2022**

The National Association of EMS Physicians and the then National Association of State EMS Directors created a position statement on emergency medical vehicle use of lights and siren in 1994. This document updates and replaces this previous statement and is now a joint position statement with the Academy of International Mobile Healthcare Integration, American Ambulance Association, American College of Emergency Physicians, Center for Patient Safety, International Academies of Emergency Dispatch, International Association of EMS Chiefs, International Association of Fire Chiefs, National Association of EMS Physicians, National Association of Emergency Medical Technicians, National Association of State EMS Officials, National EMS Management Association, National EMS Quality Alliance, National Volunteer Fire Council and Paramedic Chiefs of Canada.

In 2009, there were 1,579 ambulance crash injuries, and most EMS vehicle crashes occur when driving with lights and siren (L&S). When compared with other similar-sized vehicles, ambulance crashes are more often at intersections, more often at traffic signals, and more often with multiple injuries, including 84% involving three or more people.

From 1996 to 2012, there were 137 civilian fatalities and 228 civilian injuries resulting from fire service vehicle incidents and 64 civilian fatalities and 217 civilian injuries resulting from ambulance incidents. According to the U.S. Fire Administration (USFA), 179 firefighters died as the result of vehicle crashes from 2004 to 2013. The National EMS Memorial Service reports that approximately 97 EMS practitioners were killed in ambulance collisions from 1993 to 2010 in the United States.

Traffic-related fatality rates for law enforcement officers, firefighters, and EMS practitioners are estimated to be 2.5 to 4.8 times higher than the national average among all occupations. In a recent survey of 675 EMS practitioners, 7.7% reported being involved in an EMS vehicle crash, with 100% of those occurring in clear weather and while using L&S. Eighty percent reported a broadside strike as the type of MVC. Additionally, one survey found estimates of approximately four "wake effect" collisions (defined as collisions *caused* by, but not *involving* the L&S operating emergency vehicle) for every crash involving an emergency vehicle.

For EMS, the purpose of using L&S is to improve patient outcomes by decreasing the time to care at the scene or to arrival at a hospital for additional care, but only a small percentage of medical emergencies have better outcomes from L&S use. Over a dozen studies show that the average time saved with L&S response or transport ranges from 42 seconds to 3.8 minutes. Alternatively, L&S response increases the chance of an EMS vehicle crash by 50% and almost triples the chance of crash during patient transport (11). Emergency vehicle crashes cause delays to care and injuries to patients, EMS practitioners, and the public. These crashes also increase emergency vehicle resource use through the need for additional vehicle responses, have long-lasting effects on the reputation of an emergency organization, and increase stress and anxiety among emergency services personnel.

Despite these alarming statistics, L&S continue to be used in 74% of EMS responses, and 21.6% of EMS transports, with a wide variation in L&S use among agencies and among census districts in the United States.

Although L&S response is currently common to medical calls, few (6.9%) of these result in a potentially lifesaving intervention by emergency practitioners. Some agencies have used an evidence-based or quality improvement approach to reduce their use of L&S during responses to medical calls to 20–33%, without any discernable harmful effect on patient outcome.

Additionally, many EMS agencies transport very few patients to the hospital with L&S.

Emergency medical dispatch (EMD) protocols have been proven to safely and effectively categorize requests for medical response by type of call and level of medical acuity and urgency. Emergency response agencies have successfully used these EMD categorizations to prioritize the calls that justify an L&S response. Physician medical oversight, formal quality improvement programs, and collaboration with responding emergency services agencies to understand outcomes is essential to effective, safe, consistent, and high-quality EMD.

The sponsoring organizations of this statement (that follows) believe that the following principles should guide L&S use during emergency vehicle response to medical calls and initiatives to safely decrease the use of L&S when appropriate:

- The primary mission of the EMS system is to provide out-of-hospital health care, saving lives, and improving patient outcomes, when possible, while promoting safety and health in communities. In selected time-sensitive medical conditions, the difference in response time with L&S may improve the patient's outcome.

- EMS vehicle operations using L&S pose a significant risk to both EMS practitioners and the public. Therefore, during response to emergencies or transport of patients by EMS, L&S should only be used for situations where the time saved by L&S operations is anticipated to be clinically important to a patient's outcome. They should not be used when returning to station or posting on stand-by assignments.

- Communication centers should use EMD programs developed, maintained, and approved by national standard-setting organizations with structured call triage and call categorization to identify subsets of calls based upon response resources needed and medical urgency of the call. Active physician medical oversight is critical in developing response configurations and modes for these EMD protocols. These programs should be closely monitored by a formal quality assurance (QA) program for accurate use and response outcomes, with such QA programs being in collaboration with the EMS agency physician medical director.

- Responding emergency agencies should use response-based EMD categories and other local policies to further identify and operationalize the situations where L&S response or transport are clinically justified. Response agencies should use these dispatch categories to prioritize expected L&S response modes. The EMS agency physician medical director and QA programs must be engaged in developing these agency operational policies/guidelines.

- Emergency response agency leaderships, including physician medical oversight and QA personnel should monitor the rates of use, appropriateness, EMD protocol compliance, and medical outcomes related to L&S use during response and patient transport.

- Emergency response assignments based upon approved protocols should be developed at the local/department/agency level. A thorough community risk assessment, including risk reduction analysis, should be conducted, and used in conjunction with local physician medical oversight to develop and establish safe response policies.

- All emergency vehicle operators should successfully complete a robust initial emergency vehicle driver training program, and all operators should have required regular continuing education on emergency vehicle driving and appropriate L&S use.

- Municipal government leaders should be aware of the increased risk of crashes associated with L&S response to the public, emergency responders, and patients. Service agreements with emergency medical response agencies can mitigate this risk by using tiered response time expectations based upon EMD categorization of calls. Quality care metrics, rather than time metrics, should drive these contract agreements.

- Emergency vehicle crashes and near misses should trigger clinical and operational QA reviews. States and provinces should monitor and report on emergency medical vehicle crashes for better understanding of the use and risks of these warning devices.

- EMS and fire agency leaders should work to understand public perceptions and expectations regarding L&S use. These leaders should work toward improving public education about the risks of L&S use to create safer expectations of the public and government officials.

In most settings, L&S response or transport saves less than a few minutes during an emergency medical response, and there are few time-sensitive medical emergencies where an immediate intervention or treatment in those minutes is lifesaving. These time-sensitive emergencies can usually be identified through utilization of high-quality dispatcher call prioritization using approved EMD protocols. For many medical calls, a prompt response by EMS practitioners without L&S provides high-quality patient care without the risk of L&S-related crashes. EMS care is part of the much broader spectrum of acute health care, and efficiencies in the emergency department, operative, and hospital phases of care can compensate for any minutes lost with non-L&S response or transport.

*(continues)*

are all getting involved and generating more conversation about the issue of EMS driving safety. Chapter 7 discusses the emergency response in detail, and Chapter 3 discusses the legal elements of emergency vehicle operation.

Certainly the data available on EMS-related crashes are disconcerting, especially now, when practitioners are more conscious of safety than ever before. This is a profession that needs to be as safe as possible and injuries or deaths in the line of duty should not be an acceptable risk. Even with the increased focus on safety, there are still many human behaviors embedded in the EMS culture (e.g., lack of sleep, working additional hours to offset low wages, no licensing requirements specific to EVOs, employers "pushing" EVOs to rush so they can take the next call, etc.). These will be discussed in the following chapters.

## National EMS Memorial

Each year the National EMS Memorial Foundation conducts a service in Washington, DC, to honor those EMS practitioners who have died in the line of duty (**Figure 1-1**). The service is usually attended by family members and friends of those who are being added to the memorial. The information in **Table 1-1** is based on the lists of those honorees from the 2021, 2022, and pre-2021 historical additions. It was interesting to note that there were a significant number of additional ambulance accident deaths from pre-2021 that were added to the memorial.

## The Emergency Vehicle Operator Selection Process

A key question in the emergency vehicle operator selection process is, are we selecting only a driver or are we selecting EMTs and paramedics and training them as drivers? The latter scenario is more common. Human resources departments provide selection criteria that should be developed with plenty of input from the EMS personnel.

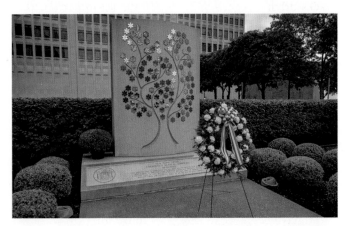

**Figure 1-1**  This is the New York State EMS Memorial in Albany. The plan is to build a National EMS Memorial in Washington, DC. In 2018, recognizing the commitment, service, and sacrifice of the lost or disabled members of the EMS practitioner community, Congress passed Public Law 115-275 authorizing the National EMS Memorial Foundation to establish a fitting and permanent National EMS Memorial in Washington, DC. The memorial is currently in the fundraising and planning phases of development.
Courtesy of the New York State Department of Health.

There are few legal restrictions on becoming an EVO; these regulations are state imposed. Unlike other professional vehicle operators, such as bus or truck drivers, whose requirements include formal training, an evaluation process to demonstrate competency, and a physical exam, the EVO's minimum requirements include age and a valid driver's license. This means that the conversation of how to keep risky or unskilled EVOs out of the driver's seat falls to individual services.

There should be focused discussions about the qualities that make a good emergency vehicle operator and should undoubtedly include such concerns as background motor vehicle operator checks, maturity, responsibility, and intrinsic motivation. Most states have a process for the department to obtain an abstract of the prospective

**Table 1-1**  Line of Duty Deaths (LODD)

| LODD as a result of | 2021 | Pre-2021 historical additions | 2022 | Total | % total |
|---|---|---|---|---|---|
| Ambulance accident | 7 | 51 | 4 | 62 | 28.7% |
| Airplane/helicopter crash | 15 | 0 | 4 | 19 | 8.8% |
| COVID-19 | 28 | 0 | 41 | 69 | 31.9% |
| Medical event | 14 | 14 | 13 | 41 | 18.9% |
| WTC certified related | 4 | 0 | 6 | 10 | 4.6% |
| Other causes | 4 | 7 | 4 | 15 | 6.9% |
| Grand total | | | | 216 | 100% |

EVO's driving record. History can be an important predictor of future behavior, and not hiring someone with a history of driving problems is important. It is also important to create a culture of safe driving in every service, in which dangerous driving and risky behaviors are unacceptable and reporting such behaviors is encouraged.

# Lessons Learned from Actual Crashes

Most crashes are reviewed by one or many agencies to determine the factors that caused the crash and ways it could have been prevented. At a minimum, the local police department and your EMS agency should investigate all crashes. At some point, once the legal dust settles, there should be a report that can be reviewed. If there is a lawsuit or the potential for one, it might be difficult to obtain copies of materials to analyze. In some instances, there may have been oversight review from an outside agency, insurance investigators, the state health department, the state or local police, the National Traffic Safety Board, and other parties, which can produce very useful reports to review and formulate, from a quality improvement perspective, the lessons we should all learn from the incident.

This text presents seven Operator Incident and six Crash Analysis boxes, along with opening Scenarios in each chapter, which have all been developed from actual crashes. This is just a starting point. The extent of the problem should become clear to you as you seriously consider the factors—mostly human factors—which led to these collisions. Some of the lessons learned from analyzing crashes have been developed into simulations so more practitioners can benefit from them.

There is tremendous value in moving these lessons into simulations to help practitioners avoid similar mistakes. Typically, simulations have been most useful in high-risk or high-cost incidents, which happen in low

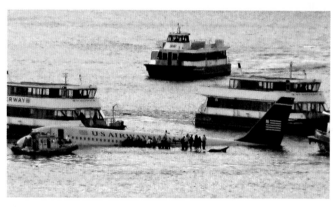

**Figure 1-2**  On January 15, 2009, Captain Chesley Burnett Sullenberger III, successfully landed U.S. Airways flight 1549 in the Hudson River off Manhattan, NY.
© Steven Day/AP Photo

frequency. In respect to driving an emergency vehicle, which is a high-frequency activity with a perceived low risk, EMS needs to move away from the idea that simulation teaches how to drive, and toward the understanding that simulation can be used to help avoid replicating choices that led to a crash. In that way, the simulation is actually being used to prevent low-frequency, high-risk, costly events. The airline industry has extensive experience with simulations, which have helped to move the fatality incidence from one per million miles to one per billion miles traveled. Today, simulation is not only considered acceptable flight training, but it also accounts for more hours of training than actual flight time. Captain Sullenberger, who was presented with a sudden in-flight emergency, had to safely glide U.S. Airways flight 1549 to a landing on the Hudson River in New York City (**Figure 1-2**). He attributed his success, and that of his crew, to the extensive training they had received, particularly flight simulations.

The EMS industry has moved slowly into simulations, particularly for driver training. Simulations are discussed in greater detail in Chapter 11.

## CRASH ANALYSIS

### Passing Out at the Wheel in Ohio

This crash involved a single-vehicle crash of a 2014 Ford E-350 Type III ambulance that occurred on the roadside of a five-lane, undivided highway. The crash occurred during the afternoon on a cloudy day with a temperature of 35°F. The posted speed limit was 50 mph and analysis of the event data recorder (EDR) reported speed revealed the ambulance was traveling 54 mph just prior to swerving and leaving the road. The vehicle was occupied by a belted 26-year-old male driver, an unbelted 49-year-old female paramedic, and a 76-year-old male patient who was restrained on the Stryker cot. The ambulance crew was conducting a nonemergency transport of a patient from one medical facility to another, and the EVO was operating the vehicle without emergency lights and siren activated. The ambulance was traveling east in the left lane when the EVO suffered a diabetic episode (hypoglycemia) and lost consciousness. He had a history of type 1 diabetes. The ambulance departed the right side of the roadway, and the front of the ambulance struck the end terminal of a blocked-out, W-beam steel guardrail and then continued down the embankment. The ambulance struck several trees and rolled end-over 180 degrees coming to rest on its wheels facing west. The EVO, who was properly restrained, remained in his seat throughout the rollover and was transported by an ambulance to the hospital where he was treated and released. The paramedic happened to be standing up at the time of the crash and was thrown about in the back of the ambulance ending up in the side stairwell with the patient partially resting on her legs. She was taken by helicopter to the trauma center and spent the night in the hospital. The paramedic stated that the three straps and shoulder straps were secured on the patient during the transport. She also stated that in order to take a BP she removed the patient's coat and the shoulder straps. During the collision and the rollover, the stretcher remained secure but the patient did slide up and partially off the stretcher. The patient sustained multiple injuries of the head and torso from contact with the hard surface of the patient compartment wall. In addition there were lower leg abrasions, an abdominal contusion, and a liver laceration. The patient was pronounced dead at the scene of the crash.

The ambulance service covers a 300-square-mile area with a population density of 614 people per square mile. They operate 18 ambulances by contract for emergency and nonemergency calls and they screen driver's records prior to employment. They also provide an 8-hour classroom driving course as well as defensive driving and an obstacle course maneuvering and on-the-job driver training. No recertifications are required.

1. How could this crash have been prevented?
2. Does your agency have a standard operating procedure (SOP) for use of all restraints on your cot?

Modified from Indiana University Transportation Research Center. (2021, July). *Special Crash Investigations: On-Site Ambulance Crash Investigation; Vehicle: 2014 Ford E-350 Type III Ambulance; Location: Ohio; Crash date: March 2018* (Report No. DOT HS 813 133). July 2021. National Highway Traffic Safety Administration. https://crashstats.nhtsa.dot.gov/Api/Public/ViewPublication/813133

## SUMMARY

- There have been, and continue to be, too many ambulance crashes in the United States resulting in injuries and fatalities.
- The NHTSA's Emergency Vehicle Operator Course (EVOC) was the first national effort to improve emergency vehicle operator education. Other programs have since joined in the effort to reduce EMS vehicle crashes.
- A brief history of EVOC and EVOC-based training programs was presented.
- The human behaviors that contribute to collisions and fatalities must be identified and changed.
- This course, EMS Vehicle Operator Safety (EVOS), presents EVO training based on current research and best practices to reduce risk and promote a culture of safety. It includes sample policies and discussions of actual crashes so that we can all learn from these tragedies.
- An important part of the development of emergency vehicle operators is the selection and educational process.

# GLOSSARY

**Ambulance Accident Prevention Seminar (AAPS)** A course launched in 1989 by the New York State Department of Health to help improve attitudes toward emergency vehicle operation.

**Centers for Disease Control and Prevention (CDC)** The government agency that works to protect American health, safety, and security from all types of diseases, including those caused by human error and preventable problems.

**Coaching the Emergency Vehicle Operator (CEVO)** An emergency vehicle operation course offered by the National Safety Council; it launched in the early 1990s and was updated to CEVO-4 in 2021.

**emergency vehicle operator (EVO)** The individual driving the emergency vehicle, generally an ambulance, who has the ability to operate it in the emergency mode (activating the lights and/or siren).

**Emergency Vehicle Driving Training (EVDT)** An emergency vehicle operation course offered by the Volunteer Fireman's Insurance Services (VFIS); it was launched in 1980 and updated in 2016.

**Emergency Vehicle Operator Course (EVOC)** A course launched in 1978 by the U.S. Department of Transportation to reduce the incidence of emergency vehicle collisions.

**EMS Vehicle Operator Safety (EVOS)** A course launched in 1989 and updated in 2023, endorsed by the NAEMT, that is designed to promote a culture of safety, prepare EVOs, and reduce the risk of driving an emergency vehicle.

**lights and siren (L&S)** The use of lights and siren sounds per policy of the agency in a presumed emergency response to the scene or transport destination.

**National Fire Protection Association (NFPA)** A standards-setting entity that develops gold standards for the fire service.

**National Highway Traffic Safety Administration (NHTSA)** An agency of the U.S. Department of Transportation responsible for ensuring safe driving conditions.

# REFERENCES

Clawson JJ, Martin RL, Cady GA, Maio RF. The wake effect: emergency vehicle-related collisions. *Prehosp Disaster Med.* 1997; 12 (4):274-277.

Drucker C, Gerberich SG, Manser MP, Alexander BH, Church TR, Ryan AD, Becic E. Factors associated with civilian drivers involved in crashes with emergency vehicles. *Accident Analysis & Prevention.* 2013; 55:116-23.

Elling, R. (1989). Dispelling myths on ambulance accidents. *Journal of Emergency Medical Services, 14*(7), 60–64.

EMS1, Fitch & Associates, & National EMS Management Association. (2022). What Paramedics Want in 2022. Retrieved from https://www.ems1.com/ems-trend-report/articles/what-paramedics-want-in-2022-4PVYVO9rHnGRwfzW/

Grant CC, Merrifield B. Analysis of ambulance crash data. The Fire Protection Research Foundation. 2011. Quincy, MA.

Indiana University Transportation Research Center. (2021, July). Special crash investigations; On-site ambulance crash investigation; Vehicle: 2014 Ford E-350 Type III Ambulance; Location: Ohio; Crash date: March 2018 (Report No. DOT HS 813 133). NHTSA.

Jarvis JL, Hamilton V, Taigman M, Brown LH. Using red lights and sirens for emergency ambulance response: How often are potentially life-saving interventions performed? Prehosp Emerg Care. 2021; 25(4): 549-555.

Kahn CA, Pirallo RG, Kuhn EM. Characteristics of fatal ambulance crashes in the United States: an 11-year retrospective analysis. Prehosp Emerg Care. 2001;5(3):261-269.

Kupas DF. Lights and siren use by emergency medical services: Above all, do no harm. National Highway Traffic Safety Administration. 2017. Retrieved from https://www.ems.gov/pdf/Lights_and_Sirens_Use_by_EMS_May_2017.pdf

Kupas DF, Zavadsky M, Burton B, et al. Joint statement on lights & siren vehicle operations on emergency medical services (EMS) responses. National Association of EMS Physicians. Published February 14, 2022. https://naemsp.org/NAEMSP/media/NAEMSP-Documents/Annual%20Meeting/2021%20MDC%20Handouts/Joint-Statement-on-Red-Light-and-Siren-Operations-with-Logos-FINAL-(003).pdf

Maguire BJ, Hunting KL, Smith GS, Levick NR. Occupational fatalities in emergency medical services: A hidden crisis. Ann Emerg Med, 2002;40: 625-632.

Maguire BJ. Transportation-related injuries and fatalities among emergency medical technicians and paramedics. Prehosp Disaster Med. 2011;26(5): 346-352. 7.

National Association of EMS Physicians. Use of warning lights and siren in emergency medical vehicle response and patient transport. *Prehosp and Disaster Med.* 1994;9(2):133-136.

National EMS Advisory Council. (2011, December). Safety Committee Final Report: Emergency Vehicle Operator Education, Training, and Safety. Retrieved from https://www.ems.gov/assets/NEMSAC_Final_Advisory_Emergency_Vehicle_Operator_Education.pdf

National Highway Traffic Safety Administration. (n.d.). Fatal Analysis Reporting System. Retrieved from ftp://ftp.nhtsa.dot.gov/FARS

National Highway Traffic Safety Administration. (n.d.). General Estimates System (GES). Retrieved from ftp://ftp.nhtsa.dot.gov/GES

National Highway Traffic Safety Administration. (2012). MMUCC Guideline: Model Minimum Uniform Crash Criteria, Fourth Edition. Retrieved from http://www-nrd.nhtsa.dot.gov/Pubs/811631.pdf

National Highway Traffic Safety Administration. (2014, April). The National Highway Traffic Safety Administration and ground ambulance crashes. Retrieved from https://www.naemt.org/Files/HealthSafety/2014%20NHTSA%20Ground%20Amublance%20Crash%20Data.pdf

National Safety Council. (n.d.). Emergency vehicles. Retrieved from https://injuryfacts.nsc.org/motor-vehicle/road-users/emergency-vehicles/

Ray AF, Kupas DF. Comparison of crashes involving ambulances with those of similar-sized vehicles. *Prehosp Emerg Care.* 2005;9(4):412-415.

Sanddal, T. L., Sanddal, N. D., Ward, N., & Stanley, L. (2010). Ambulance crash characteristics as defined by the popular press: A retrospective analysis. *Emergency Medicine International, 2010,* 525979. Retrieved from https://www.ncbi.nlm.nih.gov/pmc/articles/PMC3200082/#B2

Smith, N. (2015, September). A national perspective on ambulance crashes and safety. *EMSWorld.* Retrieved from https://www.hmpgloballearningnetwork.com/site/emsworld/article/12110600/a-national-perspective-on-ambulance-crashes-and-safety

Thomas, F. D., Graham, L. A., Wright, T. J., et al. (2019, December). Characterizing ambulance driver training in EMS systems (Report No. DOT HS 812 862). National Highway Traffic Safety Administration. Retrieved from https://www.ems.gov/assets/NHTSA_Characterizing_Ambulance_Driver_Training_in__EMS_Systems_Dec__2019.pdf

U.S. Fire Administration. Firefighter fatalities in the United States in 2013. 2014. Emmitsburg, MD.

Watanabe BL, Patterson GS, Kempema JM, Magailanes O, Brown LH. Is use of warning lights and sirens associated with increased risk of ambulance crashes? A contemporary analysis using national EMS information system (NEMSIS) data. *Ann Emerg Med.* 2019;74(1):101-109.

# CHAPTER 2

# Making Safety a Priority

## OBJECTIVES

**2.1** Discuss the importance of safety in any emergency response.

**2.2** Discuss the importance of ensuring mental preparedness by avoiding or managing fatigue, excessive emotion, stress, and any physical ailments that may inhibit decision making.

**2.3** Discuss the importance of developing a "safety-first" attitude.

**2.4** Discuss the importance of proper seatbelt placement, airbags, headrest positioning, mirror positioning, the use of a spotter, and equipment restraint.

**2.5** Explain how to secure a patient to the stretcher.

**2.6** Explain how to safely transport adult and child patients and passengers.

**2.7** Discuss how to establish a safe work zone in the event of a roadway incident.

**2.8** Explain what a traffic incident management (TIM) plan is and which agencies should be consulted when developing the plan.

**2.9** Outline the appropriate steps to respond safely to mechanical failure.

## SCENARIO

On a hot July day, a 27-year-old female emergency medical technician (EMT) died when the ambulance she was working in struck a support column for an elevated train track. The EMT had been riding unrestrained in the patient compartment while attending to a patient during a nonemergency medical transport. Since the transport was nonemergent, it is not clear whether being unrestrained was necessary to patient care.

Leading up to the collision, the crew departed the hospital with the patient at 11:56 AM. The patient had been placed supine on the cot, secured with lap-belt-type leg and hip restraints and loaded into the ambulance. The ambulance was traveling southbound without lights and siren on a two-lane city street. At approximately 12:15 PM, 1.5 miles from the hospital, the emergency vehicle operator (EVO) drifted through the northbound lane toward oncoming traffic and struck an elevated train track support column at an estimated speed of

*(continues)*

## SCENARIO (CONTINUED)

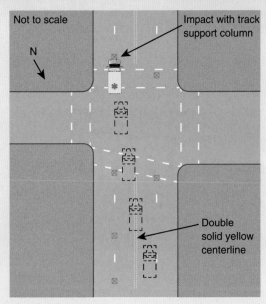

**Figure 2-1** Overhead view of the crash scene.

© Jones & Bartlett Learning

Not to scale

Impact with track support column

N

Double solid yellow centerline

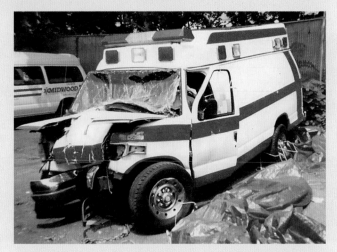

**Figure 2-2** The front/driver's side view of the damage that resulted from the ambulance striking the track support column ("El" pillar).

© Jones & Bartlett Learning. Courtesy of Rob Raheb.

26 mph (see **Figure 2-1** and **Figure 2-2**). At approximately 12:20 PM, the EVO called the office of the ambulance service to report the incident. At about the same time, witnesses called 911.

During the collision, the patient was partially ejected from the cot restraints and struck the rear-facing captain's seat at the front of the patient compartment. The EVO, who was riding unrestrained, contacted the vehicle's dash and the inflating airbag. The EMT attending to the patient impacted and broke a handrail at the end of the squad bench and struck a cabinet at the front of the patient compartment.

The EVO, EMT, and patient were transported by ambulance to a hospital. The EMT from the patient compartment was pronounced dead as a result of injuries, including a thoracic spinal cord laceration, complete cord syndrome with dislocation, bilateral lung contusions, and cerebellar subarachnoid hemorrhage.

A conclusive determination could not be made as to why the ambulance veered left across traffic and struck the support column. However, the National Automotive Sampling System (NASS) case file for this incident indicated that no avoidance maneuvers had been attempted and listed "inattentive or distracted, sleepy or fell asleep" under the category for distraction. Witnesses interviewed said that the driver admitted having no recollection of the crash.

1. Have you ever caught yourself drifting off while driving your personal vehicle or the ambulance?
2. How often do you use all available restraints for yourself and your patient?
3. Have you ever had a close call because you were not focused while driving?

## INTRODUCTION

An EMS practitioner's abilities, skills, and knowledge of emergency vehicle operation contribute to every EMS response. Every year there are millions of EMS responses that place the EMS practitioner and the general public at risk. The priority for every EMS practitioner is to ensure their own safety and the safety of their partner(s), the patient, and any passengers. Your own personal safety must be placed ahead of everyone else's. Ensuring your own safety includes being mentally and physically prepared, always fastening your seatbelt, and making sure the unit is safe to operate.

You play a key role in keeping your partner safe by ensuring the proper use of seatbelts, in both the front and the patient compartments of the ambulance. Proper safety belts are also important for patient safety, including all of the gurney shoulder straps provided by the manufacturer. The best patient care can be provided only by enforcing a "safety-first" attitude and ensuring that everyone else does the same. The right thing to do may feel uncomfortable, such as telling your partner to put on a seatbelt before you move the vehicle or asking the EVO to slow down. However, ground vehicle collisions continue to be the main cause of death for EMS practitioners, and it is important to do the right thing: Practice safety first, all the time.

# Personal Preparedness

As the operator of an emergency vehicle, you are responsible for safe vehicle operation, including the safety of the public and those in the vehicle. EVOs must be both mentally and physically prepared to perform their jobs. Mental preparation includes an awareness and management of **fatigue**, emotions, and stress while maintaining physical awareness and a safety-first attitude.

## Fatigue

Fatigue is a common cause of driver error. Most adults require 7 to 9 hours of sleep per night. Being well rested improves concentration, reaction times, and physical capabilities. Drowsy driving occurs when a person does not get the proper amount of sleep. Common signs of drowsy driving include:

- Difficulty focusing, frequent blinking, or heavy eyelids
- Daydreaming; wandering or disconnected thoughts
- Microsleeping
- Trouble remembering the last few miles driven; missing exits or traffic signs
- Yawning repeatedly or rubbing your eyes
- Trouble keeping your head up
- Drifting from your lane, tailgating, or hitting a shoulder rumble strip
- Feeling restless and irritable

It is your personal responsibility to ensure that you are well rested for your shift and are not a danger to yourself or others.

Although over 95% of Americans believe that driving while fatigued is dangerous, the numbers show that drowsy driving is a common occurrence. According to the National Sleep Foundation's (NSF) 2020 Sleep in America poll, over 60% of respondents admitted to driving when they were so tired they struggled to keep their eyes open, with 25% of drowsy drivers stating that they had done so repeatedly. A Centers for Disease Control and Prevention (CDC) survey reported that 1 in 25 adult drivers had fallen asleep while driving; sleepiness

has been implicated in over 20% of fatal motor vehicle crashes and 13% of crashes that resulted in injuries requiring hospitalization—this equals over 6,000 deaths and 100,000 injuries per year as a result of drowsy driving. Drowsy driving is even more prevalent among young drivers, with 55% of drowsy driving crashes involving drivers younger than 25 years.

Sleep deprivation and fatigue may also result in poor judgment/decision making, such as speeding. According to the NSF's poll, when asked about their behavior while driving drowsy, 42% of respondents said they become stressed, 32% said they get impatient, and 12% reported that they tend to drive faster.

Drowsy driving has been compared to another extremely dangerous and illegal practice: driving under the influence of alcohol. In the United States, a blood alcohol concentration of 0.08% is considered impaired and illegal. Studies show that being awake for 18 consecutive hours results in levels of impairment equal to those seen with a blood alcohol concentration of 0.05%; being awake for a full 24 hours produced impairment similar to a 0.096% blood alcohol concentration, which would be considered legally intoxicated in all 50 states.

Wrecks from drowsy driving can result in high personal and economic costs. Drowsy driving is believed to result in economic costs greater than $12 billion per year. Several drowsy driving incidents have resulted in jail sentences for the driver. These crashes have resulted in multimillion-dollar settlements against drivers and their companies. These costs do not include the damage to reputation and accompanying losses that a company will have due to news of the crash.

As an EVO, you are ultimately responsible for the safe operation of the vehicle. However, agencies should take precautions and create policies that ensure practitioners have the opportunity to rest before shifts. This should include mandating time off between shifts and setting maximum consecutive hours of work to prevent impairment. EMS is currently one of the very few transportation-related fields that is not regulated with mandatory time off and rest periods.

### SAFETY TIP

It is your responsibility as an EMS practitioner to ensure you are well rested, having received a recommended 7–9 hours of sleep, and fit for duty prior to the start of your shift.

## Emotions

Although emotions can be difficult to manage, EMS practitioners have a responsibility to be emotionally prepared for their shifts by not bringing personal distractions to work or allowing professional challenges to affect decision-making abilities. Any emotion, positive or negative, can affect your ability to make decisions.

Loss of control of emotions can interfere with the ability to think and focus. This lack of focus and inability to concentrate create an environment in which a driver can be distracted, affecting the ability to process information and increasing risk-taking behavior. As part of your personal preparedness, it is your responsibility to ensure that you are emotionally capable of operating an emergency vehicle. The type of run, the patient, the behavior of other drivers, and many other factors can be triggers for cumulative stress reactions. The EVO needs to be able to recognize and control those reactions when driving.

## Stress

EMS practitioners are constantly placed in high-stress environments. You must be able to properly manage your stress level and prevent it from interfering with your decision-making abilities. Stress associated with an EMS response can occur frequently and affects each individual differently. For example, your stress may increase when a call involves a pediatric patient, while another person's stress may increase when the call involves a patient with Alzheimer disease. These responses may be delayed or cumulative, manifesting in reactions to other situations.

As stress levels increase, so do levels of adrenaline and cortisol, as the body prepares for a fight-or-flight response. The increase in these stress hormones affects the vehicle operator by increasing pulse rate and elevating blood pressure. Adrenaline also causes the pupils to dilate and take in more light, increasing the field of vision.

However, as blood is redistributed from certain areas of the brain to the muscles and internal organs, peripheral vision is decreased (tunnel vision), which consequently narrows the visual field. Increased levels of stress hormones may also result in increased risky behavior and more emotional reactions, such as frustration or anger. In addition to the physical effects of adrenaline and cortisol, stress may also affect a person physically, causing gastrointestinal discomfort, headaches, or back pain. Longer-term and consistent exposure to stress can lead to memory and concentration problems, which are especially dangerous for the EVO.

At one time or another, all EMS practitioners will be adversely affected by job-related stress. It is imperative that EMS practitioners recognize stress and change their behaviors to compensate for its adverse effects. An excellent way to combat the effects of stress is to practice safe driving habits every day. During stressful events, people who have reinforced good habits with education and training are able to make better decisions. By practicing safe vehicle operations every day, you will reduce your risk during a stressful event. The key is to stay focused,

understand that other drivers will react to the presence of your emergency vehicle in a variety of ways, and remain prepared and in control when other drivers undertake erratic maneuvers. Maintaining self-control involves not internalizing others' actions and creating a new stressor.

## Attitude

A person's attitude is a key component of mental preparedness for emergency vehicle operation. *Driving is 10% knowledge, 10% skill, and 80% attitude.* Many people feel empowered and confident when they use lights and siren as the driver of an emergency vehicle. These feelings of empowerment and confidence may lead to angry and aggressive driving, which can lead vehicle operators to take chances that they would not otherwise take, jeopardizing practitioners and patients. Aggressive driving can lead to serious injury or even death. There is no excuse for aggressive driving, even when other drivers are not reacting to your approach as legally required. As a professional, it is your job to focus on your driving, be cautious, and refuse to allow emotions to guide you behind the wheel.

A related issue concerns those EVOs who feel that because they already know how to drive, there is nothing more to teach them. This type of attitude is misguided, not only because there is always more to learn, but because it is critical that EVOs know and understand the unique hazards inherent in operating an emergency vehicle. Avoiding aggressive driving and having a safety-first attitude are central to safe vehicle operation.

## Physical Awareness

Your state of health, both physical and mental, can affect your ability to operate an emergency vehicle. Therefore, physical awareness is an important part of ensuring your preparedness and safety. Physical awareness includes being sensitive to any health problems. It is also important to remember that over-the-counter (OTC) treatments can affect physical awareness and the ability to react and respond to emergencies, not to mention the dangers of operating a vehicle while under the influence of alcohol or other drugs. The following are some examples of physical disruptions that could affect your performance:

- A leg sprain or strain may cause difficulty in moving your foot from the accelerator to the brake, thus delaying reaction time.
- Gastrointestinal distress may cause you to become less focused and attentive to detail or to rush your actions.
- A cold or flu may be associated with distracting symptoms such as a runny nose, which can lead to loss of focus.
- Headaches, especially migraine headaches, may cause changes in vision and hearing, which can severely diminish your ability to operate an emergency vehicle.

# Safety Equipment

Emergency vehicles are equipped with safety equipment, such as seatbelts and airbags. Proper use of this equipment is essential to ensure the safety of the EVO, EMS practitioners, and the patients they transport. The most important safety device in the vehicle is the EVO. By remaining alert and calm, and recognizing potential hazards before they occur, the EVO can be the difference between crashing and avoiding a collision.

## Seatbelts

Seatbelts are an extremely effective method of reducing injuries and deaths from vehicle collisions. Over 15,000 lives are saved each year by proper use of seatbelts, and most EMS organizations have polices requiring the use of seatbelts in emergency vehicles.

The National Highway Traffic Safety Administration's (NHTSA's) Special Crash Investigations teams conduct investigations of serious ambulance crashes. One analysis of over 50 of these incidents revealed a startling fact: EMS personnel are not buckling up! The analysis revealed that, at the time of the crash, over 80% of EMS practitioners in the back of the ambulance were unbelted and over 20% of EVOs in the passenger compartment were not wearing restraints. There is absolutely no excuse for this risky behavior; all agencies should have a clear seatbelt standard operating procedure (SOP) and should consider the use of "black box" technology to track seatbelt use.

For seatbelts to be effective, they must be worn properly. The lap belt needs to be placed snugly over the hips. The shoulder belt should be placed over the shoulder and diagonally across the torso away from the neck as shown in **Figure 2-3**. The shoulder belt should never be placed under the arm. Shorter or taller individuals may need to adjust the seatbelt restraint system or the position of the seat to ensure that the seatbelt fits properly. In older vehicles with separate lap and shoulder restraints, both systems must be used. Wearing a safety belt improperly may increase the risk of injury to a level similar to that of not wearing a seatbelt at all.

Although the evidence is overwhelming that seatbelts save lives, many people still do not wear them, including people working in EMS. Practitioners may think it is acceptable to stand or move around unrestrained in the patient compartment when the vehicle is in motion. Even those who have witnessed the often tragic consequences of not wearing a seatbelt may rationalize this practice, but unrestrained practitioners providing patient care are at significant risk for injury and death in the event of a collision.

As the EVO, you are responsible for ensuring that everyone is wearing a seatbelt properly before moving the vehicle. This includes practitioners in the patient

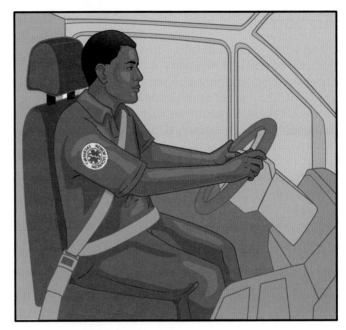

**Figure 2-3** Proper seatbelt use.
© Jones & Bartlett Learning

compartment. Unrestrained or improperly restrained EMS practitioners die or are seriously injured each year in motor vehicle collisions. Even though it is legal, it is not safe practice for EMS practitioners to be unrestrained, even when providing patient care.

> **SAFETY TIP**
>
> The single most important factor in seatbelt use is personal commitment. Make a commitment to always ensure your safety first.

It may be more difficult or inconvenient to provide patient care while wearing a seatbelt, but this is no excuse to not wear one. Research is under way to develop a more ergonomic work space that will allow practitioners to tend to patients while being restrained. Regardless of the system in place, the EVO must be properly restrained and ensure that all crew members are wearing seatbelts. This simple step can mean the difference between minor injury and death in the event of a motor vehicle collision. Recommendations for developing a SOP for seatbelt use in the ambulance are included in Chapter 12.

> **SAFETY TIP**
>
> Seatbelts save lives. There is no excuse for not using seatbelts in the front compartment. Moreover, they should be used in the patient compartment.

## Airbags

Airbags are important safety features that help to reduce **morbidity** and **mortality** in the event of a collision. Frontal airbags in emergency vehicles are usually located in the steering wheel or the dashboard and are designed to protect the occupant from hitting the steering wheel, dashboard, and windshield. Newer ambulances may include other types of airbags such as side curtain airbags, rollover airbags, knee bolsters, carpet airbags, and/or antislide airbags.

Vehicle occupants should be a safe distance from the airbag (at least 10 in). No objects, including mobile data terminals or other devices, should obstruct the path between the occupant and the airbag. Objects located in this path during airbag deployment could interfere with the release of the airbag or become projectiles and cause further injury. It is important to remember that airbags are only part of the occupant safety system and that proper seatbelt use is required as well. Newer model vehicles will not deploy the airbag if the seat belt is not utilized. Data from the CDC show that seat belts with airbags reduce the risk of death by 45% and injury by 50%.

## Headrests or Head Restraints

Head restraints, more commonly called headrests, in emergency vehicles vary depending on the make, model, and year of the vehicle. When available, they may help to reduce neck injuries in the event of a rear-end collision. Many drivers have improperly adjusted head restraints, the most common error being that the head restraints are adjusted too low. A head restraint should be positioned no more than 2 in behind the driver's head, with the center of the headrest at approximately ear level. When adjusted properly, the driver's head should contact the head restraint before the neck does (**Figure 2-4**).

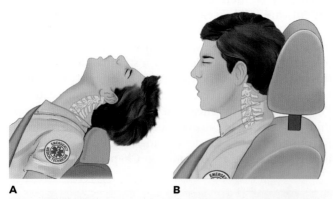

**A**          **B**

**Figure 2-4** **A.** If a headrest is improperly positioned, the head can be hyperextended over the top of the headrest during a rear-impact collision, causing injury. **B.** If a headrest is properly positioned, neck injury is prevented or reduced during collision.
© National Association of Emergency Medical Technicians (NAEMT)

Properly positioning the head restraint may reduce whiplash and other neck injuries in the event of a rear-end collision.

## Mirrors

Properly adjusted mirrors are important to safe vehicle operation. It is the EVO's responsibility to ensure the mirrors are positioned to maximize the operator's field of vision and limit blind spots. Mirrors may need to be adjusted multiple times during a shift in situations where drivers change frequently. Mirrors should be adjusted following the one-fifth, one-third rule: Adjust the mirrors so that your vehicle occupies one-fifth of the inside vertical portion of the mirror and the horizon is seen in the top one-third of the mirror. Setting mirrors in this fashion gives every driver the largest field of view. By simply leaning forward, the EVO can increase the field of view and reduce blind spots around the vehicle.

It is important to remember that even when you have properly maximized your field of vision, blind spots are still present behind the vehicle. To back the vehicle safely, use a spotter to provide directions. Services should have strict policies requiring use of a spotter when backing a vehicle. Recommended backing protocols can be found in Chapter 12.

> **SAFETY TIP**
>
> Being safe is a personal commitment and is a *must* for every EVO. Be committed to your safety and the safety of others.

## Equipment Security

Properly securing equipment is essential to prevent it from becoming a projectile during a collision or sudden stop. Unsecured equipment such as first-in bags (jump kits), oxygen caddies, defibrillators, or monitors may become deadly projectiles and have been documented to cause practitioner and patient injury. Equipment should always be secured in cabinets or in specifically designed locations. One method of securing gear is to attach a properly rated and approved carabiner to the bag (jump kit) and clip it to a specified location in the box. Properly securing equipment takes only a few seconds; there is simply no justifiable reason to leave equipment unsecured. Ambulances should be properly equipped with monitor locks and computer docking stations to secure equipment in a usable position.

## Helmets

When an ambulance is involved in a collision or evasive maneuver, unrestrained practitioners may fall and strike their heads. Unrestrained equipment such as oxygen gauges or suction unit bottles may become airborne and strike practitioners, and sharp corners or edges may cause injuries. Thus, some safety experts advocate the use of safety helmets for EMS personnel during patient transport.

Dr. Nadine Levick, CEO of Objective Safety and Research Director of EMS Safety Foundation, reports that 74% of EMS fatalities are the result of vehicle collisions and that 64% of those deaths are the result of serious head injuries. It is logical to presume that helmets could help reduce morbidity and mortality in these situations. Specially designed helmets for protecting EMS personnel have yet to be developed, and traditional fire helmets would not be effective for this purpose. The use of helmets, however, would not reduce the need to improve ambulance design and testing for greater safety or the use of other safety procedures (use of restraints, properly securing equipment, etc.). Routine helmet use will require further education, training, positive reinforcement, and practical policies implemented by visionary leaders who are committed to safety and research.

> **SAFETY TIP**
>
> Gear should always be secured in a compartment or specified location.

# Patient Safety

When patients call 911 requesting an ambulance, they expect to be transported safely. Remember rule number one: Do no harm. You should never put a patient in jeopardy during transport.

One essential way to ensure patient safety is through proper use of stretcher restraints. Additional data from the NHTSA's Special Crash Investigations study show that while 96% of patients were restrained with lateral belts at the time of a crash, only 33% were fully secured to the cot with shoulder straps. Many practitioners assume that when a patient is secured on the stretcher with three lateral belts and the stretcher is properly latched to the floor, the patient is safe. Unfortunately, this is not true. Use of lateral straps alone significantly increases the risk of patients being ejected from the cot in the event of a crash, and ejection is related to an increased risk of fatal injuries.

Patients should always be secured to the stretcher using a four-point shoulder harness with a chest strap, a pelvis strap, and a leg strap (**Figure 2-5**). Stretcher manufacturers now generally include a four-point shoulder harness as part of their standard equipment. Many practitioners believe that the shoulder harnesses are optional, but in fact, they are critical for ensuring that the patient does not slide out of the stretcher straps during a

collision. It is imperative that practitioners use the manufacturer's specifications for securing patients; failure to do so could result in increased liability for injuries in the case of a collision. The scenario at the beginning of this chapter is a good example. When the shoulder harnesses are properly secured in accordance with the manufacturer's recommendations, they should not interfere with your ability to provide patient care, including a 12-lead electrocardiogram (ECG) or other monitoring.

> **SAFETY TIP**
>
> You have the responsibility to ensure that your patients are properly secured. In many instances, patients who were improperly secured (without the use of the provided shoulder harnesses) have been killed or severely injured following a vehicle collision. Your patient's safety is your responsibility.

The stretcher should be secured to the floor during transport. Slightly raise the head end to help prevent the patient from hitting the captain's seat or bulkhead in the event of a frontal impact crash. Note, however, that even when properly secured, ambulance crash tests have revealed that stretchers can detach from the mounts and become projectiles in the event of a collision. It is interesting to note that in the United States, the locking system of the most commonly used stretchers and mounting systems is designed to withstand only 2,200 foot-pounds of force—roughly equivalent to only 74 pounds moving at 30 mph. In addition, stretchers are secured at only a single point of contact on a rack that prevents the wheels from rolling too far forward. In comparison, stretchers

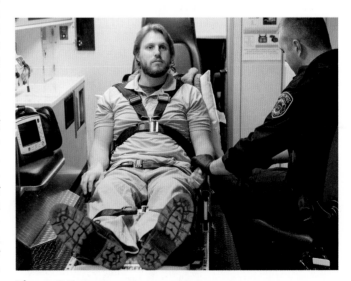

**Figure 2-5** Proper patient restraints.
© Jones & Bartlett Learning. Photographed by Darren Stahlman.

used in Europe and their mounting systems are able to endure loads 10 times the force of gravity over a crash impulse window of less than 100 milliseconds without failure. Further, stretchers are secured to the floor at three points of contact, each of which restrains motion on at least two axes.

# Passenger Safety

Family members and friends often want to accompany patients in the ambulance. Your company should have a policy for these cases, and you should be familiar with the policy to ensure that this is an approved practice.

An adult passenger should be transported in the front passenger seat and wear a seatbelt. The EVO should assist the passenger into the front seat and ensure that the seatbelt is properly attached. The EVO should also assist the passenger out of the vehicle upon arrival at the destination. Any passenger who refuses to wear a seatbelt should not be permitted to ride in the ambulance. Small folding stools may be useful to help passengers into and out of the passenger seat. These stools may be stored behind the passenger seat of the ambulance.

EVOs should not allow themselves to become distracted by conversing with accompanying family members or friends. The primary objective is getting to the hospital safely, and this may require the operator's full attention. It is not discourteous to inform passengers that you are unable to talk while driving to ensure that everyone arrives safely at their destination.

While in general, passengers should be seated in the front compartment, there are certain circumstances in which it may be advantageous for a passenger to ride in the patient compartment. For example, it may be beneficial for a parent to ride in the patient compartment to provide support to a pediatric patient. In this event, the child must be properly restrained in accordance with their age and size and with local laws. Children should never be transported on the parent's lap, even if the parent is secured to the stretcher. Parents in the patient compartment must also be properly restrained.

Prior to allowing the parent to ride with the patient, a member of the crew should explain any necessary interventions so that the parent knows what to expect during transport. Parents who are overly emotional or unable to

> **SAFETY TIP**
>
> EMS practitioners should never sit on the end of the stretcher to provide patient care during transport. This practice places the patient at risk of being injured by the practitioner should a vehicle collision occur.

control themselves should not be permitted to ride in the patient compartment. Family members or friends should never be transported in the patient compartment when the patient is in respiratory or cardiac arrest or when other critical conditions exist.

In special situations, children may need to be transported as passengers when their parent is a patient. This practice should be limited to situations in which no other options exist. Children who are eligible to ride in the passenger seat according to your state law should ride in the passenger seat with proper restraints. Children who require a safety seat must be transported in a child safety seat or booster seat. Safety seats may not be placed on side-facing seats. Children who are not required to use a child safety seat of any kind may ride in the captain's seat (rear-facing seat) with a seatbelt, based on your department's policy.

When necessary, additional emergency responders may be transported as passengers. It is the responsibility of the EVO to ensure that they are properly restrained the same as any other crew member. Remember that the number of occupants should never exceed the number of seatbelts in the vehicle.

> **SAFETY TIP**
>
> If the patient is not in a critical condition that requires immediate hospital resources, the transport should be considered nonemergent and the EVO should drive accordingly with the crew and patient properly restrained at all times. If the patient requires immediate transportation to the hospital due to their condition and the crew is unable to remain seatbelted due to the need to provide patient care, the EVO should slow down and give as smooth a ride as possible.

# Roadside Safety

Many emergency incidents occur on interstates, highways, and other roadways. An emergency scene on the roadway presents unique hazards to emergency responders of all types. In 2022, 51 responders (including 11 from fire/EMS) were killed after being struck by another vehicle.

Motorists may be distracted by the scene and not paying attention to their driving. Because our hands follow our eyes, we tend to drive in the direction in which we are looking; motorists looking at an accident scene (instead of straight ahead) may veer toward the accident unintentionally. The safest place for an emergency vehicle responding to a highway incident is off of the roadway and away from traffic. EVOs need to ensure they are

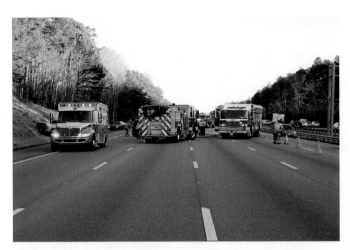

**Figure 2-6** Proper traffic blocking techniques and high-visibility gear will help to keep you safe.
© Mike Legeros. Used with permission.

seen by other motorists and have been given the right of way. Whenever possible, you should avoid working on a roadway or highway or at least aim to limit the amount of time you spend on the roadway as much as possible, even if it means delaying patient care until you can move to a safe location. When it is necessary to work on a roadway, you should take proper precautions:

- Establish a safe work zone by having the police or fire department block traffic and using traffic-control devices (**Figure 2-6**).
- Position the vehicle properly ("downstream" of the collision).
- Consider the use of warning lights.
- Wear high-visibility apparel that meets federal standards.

## Safe Work Zone

The answer to developing a safe work zone on the highway requires more than "Move Over Laws" or wearing high-visibility vests. A scene is always evolving and emergency personnel must be taught that safety is an ongoing process from dispatch to completion of the call. All EVOs and EMS practitioners must practice situational awareness at all times.

Emergency vehicles can be positioned to establish a safe work zone by blocking traffic and providing protection for personnel operating at the emergency scene. The key is having the first-arriving unit block traffic from the scene. Ideally, fire apparatus should be used to block traffic, but the ambulance can be used to perform this function if it is needed to secure the scene and warn oncoming drivers. The preferred placement of the ambulance is beyond (downstream) and to the side of the collision, away from the flow of traffic, which limits exposure to

moving traffic during patient loading. It is also the best position for egress once it is time to transport the patient. Cones and traffic warning devices should be used to alert motorists at extended incidents whenever possible.

If an ambulance is being used to block traffic, angle the vehicle so that it is aimed away from the scene, with the rear doors not directly facing on-coming traffic. Keep the rear doors closed so that the vehicle's lights are visible. This positioning provides additional protection so that practitioners can access equipment. In addition, turn the vehicle's wheels away from the work zone so that in the event it is struck by a motorist from behind, it will not directly collide with the scene. Note that the patient should not be loaded into the vehicle until it is moved around the incident and positioned such that the collision scene serves as a protective barrier.

At high-risk incidents and locations, it may be necessary to request assistance from additional responders (e.g., police, fire, other EMS, and highway services) to ensure scene safety. The Traffic Incident Management (TIM) system can help responders coordinate their efforts when more than one response vehicle is necessary at an incident to avoid placing the ambulance in an area that may be blocked by other emergency vehicles.

The TIM system comprises several components that both allow traffic to move safely and smoothly around an emergency scene and allow the first responders to work in a relatively safe environment. It is used to create a **temporary traffic control zone**, which includes the following areas as listed in **Figure 2-7**.

- *Advanced warning area*. This area gives approaching motorists ample warning of an incident ahead and the opportunity to transition from normal driving status to that required by the temporary emergency traffic control measures. It is usually marked with a *pink* diamond-shaped warning sign placed by the first unit arriving on scene (**Figure 2-8**). These signs are made for easy storage and quick deployment upon arrival at the scene.
- *Transition area*. This area begins the flare or cone pattern, which is used to taper the number of lanes and move traffic away from the incident. (Note: Flares should NOT be used at scenes with spilled gasoline or other flammable liquids.) A flare pattern should start approximately 50 feet from the incident, and a flare should be placed every 50 feet until all flares (usually at least six) are in position, tapering from the incident to the shoulder and guiding upstream traffic away from the incident. Consider extending this distance on curves or hills to ensure your safety. *Stay alert! Placing flares is an extremely dangerous, but important, process for helping to secure the scene.*

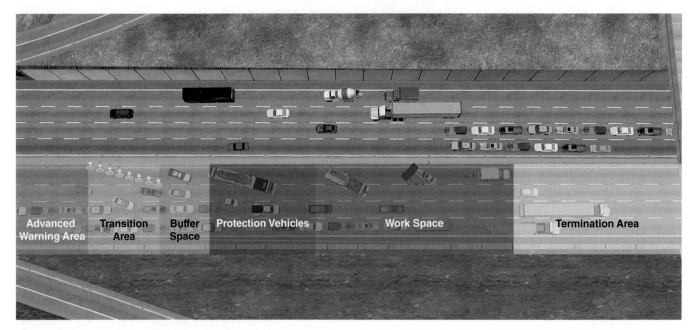

**Figure 2-7** The Traffic Incident Management (TIM) system.
Courtesy of FAAC, Inc. Based on original figure by Emergency Responder Safety Institute.

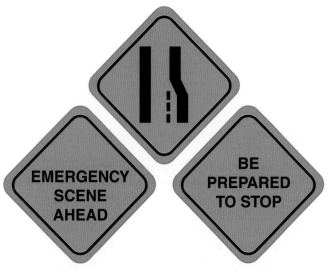

**Figure 2-8** Advanced warning area signs.
Reproduced from Federal Highway Administration. *Field Operations Guide for Safety/ Service Patrols.* U.S. Department of Transportation. December 2009. https://ops.fhwa .dot.gov/publications/fhwahop10014/fhwahop10014.pdf

- ***Buffer space***. This area starts to slow traffic and funnel it away from the incident. Law enforcement vehicles may be placed here to provide additional visual cues for motorists to move over.
- *Protection vehicles*. This area is directly upstream from the incident. Vehicles positioned here are primarily used for blocking and secondarily used as resource vehicles. Lane plus one blocking and linear positioning afford a good work space for rescuers and a "shadow" area that limits drivers' ability to rubberneck. Position vehicles to both block and direct traffic.
- *Work space*. This is the area of the incident, and it must remain as open and as safe as possible. Protection vehicles may have to be repositioned as the operation progresses to maintain a high level of safety while allowing traffic to flow with as little impediment as possible.

> **SAFETY TIP**
>
> It's usually difficult to determine what 300 feet of distance is. A good rule of thumb is that most "skip line" segments (each component of the dashed line that divides a roadway into lanes of opposing traffic) are 30 feet long. A segment constitutes the beginning of the line and the space between lines to the beginning of the next line.

> **SAFETY TIP**
>
> The number of lanes to close should be based on traffic conditions. Generally speaking, more lanes should be closed if traffic is light and/or moving quickly, and fewer lanes if traffic is already congested and moving well below the speed limit. Use good judgment; tempers run high when stuck in traffic. *Stay alert!*

- *Termination area.* This is the area immediately downstream of the incident that allows traffic to continue to move in a controlled manner. This area should be avoided by responders at all times and at all costs. If the incident dictates that responders enter into the termination area, then the work space should be extended and the termination area moved further downstream. This area can be used for staging of tow trucks, medical examiner vehicles, and other ancillary vehicles that are not actively engaged in the rescue process.

Additional concepts related to the use of the TIM system include the following:

- **Block.** Blocking involves positioning a fire department apparatus on an angle to the lanes of traffic to create a physical barrier between upstream traffic and the work area. The position of the emergency vehicle subconsciously diverts the motorist in the direction that steers them away from the incident, so be sure to block to the left when on the outside shoulder or to the right of the center lane and block to the right when on the inside shoulder or left of the center lane. If the incident is in the middle of the roadway, consider shutting the roadway down or blocking off the road from the inside shoulder and divert all traffic toward the right of the incident. *Do not allow traffic to travel around both sides of the incident.*
- **Downstream.** In regard to the direction of travel, the area after the incident, where traffic is moving away from the incident.
- *Lane plus one blocking.* Positioning a fire department apparatus in a manner that blocks the incident lane and one additional lane from approaching traffic.
- **Linear.** Positioning a vehicle within or parallel to a lane of travel or shoulder to protect the incident scene and visibly shield the scene from passing drivers. This provides a barrier only in the lane or shoulder in which the vehicle is parked and does little to funnel traffic; should be used in conjunction with block positioning.
- **Taper.** Direct traffic to merge into adjacent lanes for the purposes of reducing the number of active travel lanes. This is initiated in the transition area and is completed in the buffer space.
- **Upstream.** In regard to the direction of travel, the area before the incident, where traffic is moving toward the incident.

Become familiar with the TIM system. If you have any questions about vehicle placement at an incident, consult with the incident commander, who has overall responsibility for scene safety and comprehensive

knowledge about the operations. For more in-depth information regarding the TIM system, visit the Emergency Responder Safety Institute website.

## Vehicle Positioning

It is important to position the emergency vehicle properly at an emergency scene to ensure the safety of motorists, patients, and practitioners. Consider the location of the incident and unique hazards, such as inclement weather and poor visibility, when determining the safest places to position the vehicle. For example, vehicles should not be placed on corners, at the crest of hills, or in blind spots. EVOs need to be aware of the unique hazards within their response district.

When staging the vehicle at a scene, several issues may need to be taken into account in the placement of the vehicle, not only for safe scene operations but also for easy egress once scene management is complete. Examples include placing vehicles uphill from spilled liquids and vapors, upwind from fumes and smoke, upstream when first on scene, and downstream when on scene with other units and loading patients. Vigilance should be used when positioning the ambulance so as not to get blocked in by additional emergency vehicles, prohibiting rapid transport from the scene.

Many emergency responses occur at a residence or other location where there is a driveway. In these instances, the driveway is usually the safest place to park the ambulance. When arriving at the incident location, depending on the situation and priority of the assignment, your partner should exit the vehicle wearing high-visibility apparel and serve as a spotter to help you back into the driveway. When the vehicle is on the street, the EVO can take command of the roadway and can control the flow of traffic when backing into a location.

Backing in allows the EVO to easily leave the scene, as they can see cross traffic before entering the roadway; this is especially helpful because your partner is likely tending to the patient and may not be able to spot you while backing into traffic. In some situations, it may be necessary to park at the curb in front of the residence. Either way, once the vehicle is parked, the emergency lights and headlights should be turned off if they might interfere with the normal flow of traffic in any way.

---

**OPERATOR INCIDENT**

In southwestern Colorado on a March day, several teenagers were killed due to improper parking and misuse of warning equipment by an EVO at the scene. A deputy investigating a car off the road drove past a collision on a curve and parked without using emergency lights, leaving his headlights on. The deputy parked to the right of the travel lanes and left of the disabled vehicle. This created an optical illusion with the stopped car, creating the appearance that the oncoming lane was further right than it really was. As a result, the fatigued driver of an oncoming utility truck drove into the scene on the shoulder, striking the teenagers inside of and around the disabled vehicle. The truck driver saw the deputy's headlights and mistakenly thought the deputy was in the approaching lane. Had the deputy used his emergency lights, turned off the headlights, or lit the scene properly, this incident may have been avoided.

---

## Warning Lights

It may seem counterintuitive, but emergency lights may actually be a safety hazard. It is not uncommon for motorists to crash into parked emergency vehicles that have warning lights operating, and these secondary crashes are a leading cause of death for emergency responders.

Given the wide range of options for emergency lighting configurations, in 2021, the Emergency Responder Safety Institute's study, Effects of Emergency Vehicle Lighting Characteristics on Driver Perception and Behavior, investigated the impact of lighting color, intensity, modulation, and flash rate on driver responses to an incident at night. The study authors made the following recommendations:

- Higher intensity does not equal better visibility. At night, lower intensity lights provide essentially the same level of visibility as those of higher intensity, with less glare. As such, reduced intensity lights should be used with stationary vehicles in blocking mode at nighttime incidents.
- The color of the light affects its perceived brightness. At the same intensity, drivers judged blue and red lights as brighter than white and yellow lights.

Red lights were also judged as producing the least amount of glare. These findings suggest that red lights may be ideal for stationary blocking operations.

- Current minimum intensity requirements (e.g., NFPA 1901, *Standard for Automotive Fire Apparatus*) for flashing lights on emergency vehicles, while appropriate for daytime operations, may be brighter than needed for use at night for stationary vehicles. Lower intensity lights (below minimum requirements) were still rated as highly visible, with the added benefit of reduced glare and driver discomfort.
- Concerns about motorists driving toward flashing lights appear to be unfounded. No "moth-to-flame" effect (or its opposite) was seen in any of the studies; neither intensity nor color had any effect on how close participants drove to the lights. (As discussed earlier, drivers may drift toward accident scenes as a result of looking at the accident instead of the road ahead of them, but this is unrelated to the use of lights on scene.)
- High-reflectivity materials, in combination with high-intensity lights, seem to negatively impact a driver's ability to see responders at the incident scene, even if the responders are wearing safety vests. When highly reflective materials were used to simulate the chevrons on the back of fire apparatus with flashing lights, the average distance at which participants could discern the silhouette of a nearby responder was less than when lower-intensity lights were used. This suggests that less-reflective materials may be preferable for marking the rear of fire apparatus, rather than higher types.

In addition, most newer vehicles have "scene activation" lighting that automatically dims or shuts off certain lights when the vehicle is placed into park. Not all vehicles are equipped with this feature and it is not a mandatory standard. As always, familiarize yourself with your agency's equipment and follow local SOPs.

The use of warning lights for blocking vehicles is discussed in detail in NFPA 1451, *Standard for a Fire and Emergency Service Vehicle Operations Training Program*.

## High-Visibility Apparel

High-visibility apparel increases the practitioner's visibility when working along a roadway. Federal law requires all workers within the right of way along a federal highway to wear an ANSI 107 (2004) Class 2 or 3 high-visibility vest. This law applies to all first responders, though exceptions do exist for police personnel based on tactical need. The use of high-visibility vests increases personnel visibility and reduces the risk of severe injury or death (**Figure 2-9**). These vests are also required to come with a five-point breakaway feature for safety. However, it is important to understand that the use of high-visibility apparel alone does not make you safe.

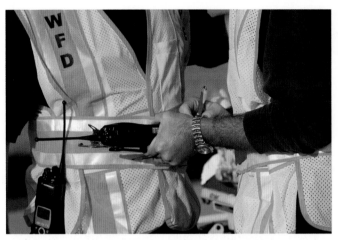

**Figure 2-9** Agencies should obtain high-visibility vests (ANSI-107 [2004] Class 2 or 3 garments or ANSI-207 [2006]-compliant garments) for their personnel. Ensure that vests are sized to fit when worn on top of full turnout gear, such as in cold-weather situations, responses to motor vehicle crashes where there is no fire, or where otherwise appropriate.

© Nancy G Fire Photography, Nancy Greifenhagen/Alamy Stock Photo.

> **SAFETY TIP**
>
> Place approved high-visibility apparel in an easily accessible location. Use positive reinforcement and lead by example so that wearing high-visibility apparel becomes the norm.

# Mechanical Problems

As an EVO, you may encounter situations that involve safety hazards such as a mechanical problem or vehicle fire. In these situations, the overriding concern should be your personal safety and the safety of your partner, patient, and passengers.

Common mechanical problems such as engine failure, transmission failure, an overheating vehicle, or a flat tire can create an unexpected and hazardous situation. When a mechanical problem occurs, every attempt should be made to move the vehicle away from traffic. If your vehicle is blocking traffic in any way, immediately turn on your hazard lights to warn oncoming motorists. Do not use your emergency lights, as this may confuse drivers who associate the emergency lights with an incident such as a motor vehicle collision. After turning on your hazard lights, you should request assistance to control the traffic hazard in accordance with your agency's policies. Remember to request an additional unit to transport your patient, if necessary.

> **SAFETY TIP**
>
> Take precautions to protect yourself in the event of mechanical difficulties:
> - Move the vehicle away from traffic.
> - Put on the vehicle's hazard lights.
> - Call for assistance.
> - Safely exit the vehicle.
> - Use traffic-control devices.

Once assistance has been requested, you should don high-visibility apparel and exit the vehicle. To provide additional protection and warn oncoming traffic, you should set up flares, warning triangles, or other traffic-control devices. Whenever possible, place warning devices to direct traffic away from the disabled vehicle, as discussed previously. Roadside repairs should never be attempted by nonqualified personnel; always defer to local policies. Keep in mind that flares may create additional danger if there are leaking fluids on the ground.

Although rare, vehicle fires can occur in an emergency medical vehicle. Emergency medical units carry oxygen, which is an accelerant and can be extremely dangerous in the event of a fire. If a vehicle fire occurs, you must rapidly assess the situation and take actions to maximize safety. The priority should be removing the patient from the vehicle. If the vehicle is on fire, you should not take time to remove equipment. Since the oxygen system on board could result in an explosion, your main concern is to move yourself and the patient a safe distance away from the vehicle.

## CRASH ANALYSIS

### Ambulance Fire in Hawaii

Though not a crash, this incident involved a fire in the back of an ambulance during the summer of 2022. The fire killed a 91-year old patient and injured a 36-year-old paramedic. The injured paramedic reported hearing a loud "pop" while connecting a continuous positive airway pressure (CPAP) oxygen line to a portable oxygen cylinder, followed by a bright flash of light with the back of the ambulance immediately filling with smoke and fire. The EVO reported hearing the same "pop" sound before the fire began. The origin of the fire was found to be the portable oxygen cylinder regulator assembly. Possible causes may include contamination or particles in the oxygen cylinder, but an exact cause was not determined. The ambulance was parked at the time of the incident.

1. How could this fire have been prevented?
2. Does your agency have an SOP for providing oxygen?

## SUMMARY

- The priority for EMS practitioners is to ensure their own safety, followed by the safety of their partner, patients, and passengers.
- Having a safety-first attitude is a critical component of safe vehicle operation.
- Safety must become a habit and a culture that relies on personal responsibility and commitment to excellence.
- Mental and physical preparedness includes efforts to reduce or avoid fatigue, stress, extreme emotions, or physical ailments, all of which may inhibit decision making.
- To be effective, a seatbelt must be placed properly, with the lap belt snug over the hips and the shoulder belt over the shoulder and diagonally across the torso.
- EMS practitioners must always be properly restrained during transport, even when they are providing care to the patient in the patient compartment.
- Emergency vehicle airbags located in the steering wheel or dashboard are designed to protect the driver and front passenger in the event of a collision.

- Properly positioned headrests can reduce the risk of neck injuries.
- Correct mirror positioning and use of spotters when backing are important safety precautions.
- It is necessary to secure all equipment to avoid projectiles if the vehicle stops suddenly.
- Patients should always be secured to the stretcher using a four-point shoulder harness with chest strap, pelvis strap, and leg strap.
- Adult passengers should ride in the front passenger seat with a seatbelt.
- Children should always be properly restrained according to their age, size, and weight in accordance with state guidelines.
- To establish a safe work zone in the event of a roadway incident, position the vehicle properly, consider the use of warning lights, and wear high-visibility apparel.
- In the event of a mechanical failure, move the vehicle away from traffic, use hazard lights, call for assistance, safely exit the vehicle, and use traffic-control devices.

## GLOSSARY

**advanced warning area** Area established to warn motorists of an approaching incident and allow them to prepare for the new traffic control pattern.

**block** To position a fire department apparatus on an angle to the lanes of traffic, creating a physical barrier between upstream traffic and the work area. Includes block to the left and block to the right.

**buffer space** The area immediately after the transition area, in which the traffic begins to slow down and move out of the incident lane.

**downstream** In regard to the direction of travel, the area after the incident, where traffic is moving away from the incident.

**fatigue** The state of having insufficient sleep.

**linear** Positioning a vehicle within or parallel to a lane of travel or shoulder to protect the incident scene. This provides a barrier only in the lane or shoulder in which the vehicle is parked and does little to funnel traffic; should be used in conjunction with block positioning.

**morbidity** Illness or harm; a diseased state.

**mortality** Death; the quality of being mortal.

**taper** To direct traffic to merge into adjacent lanes for the purposes of reducing the number of active travel lanes.

**temporary traffic control zone** An area of a roadway where normal traffic patterns have been temporarily changed; this can be due to an emergency incident, construction, special events, or maintenance of nearby structures (telephone lines, streetlights, etc.).

**transition area** The space after the advanced warning area in which the traffic changes are implemented; warning devices are placed to direct motorists out of the incident lane(s) and into the new lanes of travel. Also known as the transition zone.

**upstream** In regard to the direction of travel, the area before the incident, where traffic is moving toward the incident.

# ADDITIONAL RESOURCES

Emergency Responder Safety Institute, http://www.responder safety.com

National Fire Protection Association. (2013). *NFPA 1451: Standard for a fire and emergency services vehicle operations training program*. Quincy, MA.

National Highway Traffic Safety Administration, http://www.nhtsa.gov

National Institute of Occupational Safety and Health and Department of Homeland Security Science and Technology Directorate. *Improving EMS worker safety through ambulance design and testing* video series. www.cdc.gov/niosh/topics/ems/videos.html

National Safety Council, http://www.nsc.org

Proudfoot, S. L. (2005). Ambulance crashes: Fatality factors for EMS workers. *EMS World*. Retrieved from https://www.hmpglobal learningnetwork.com/site/emsworld/article/10323905/ambulance-crashes-fatality-factors-ems-workers

U.S. Department of Homeland Security Science and Technology Directorate, First Responders Group. (2015). *Ambulance patient compartment human factors design guidebook*. Retrieved from https://www.dhs.gov/sites/default/files/publications/Ambulance%20Patient%20Compartment%20Human%20Factors%20Design%20Guidebook.pdf

U.S. Department of Labor, Occupational Safety and Health Administration (OSHA), http://www.osha.gov

U.S. Department of Transportation, Federal Highway Administration. *Manual on Uniform Traffic Control Devices for Streets and Highways*, 2009 Edition (including Revision 1–May 2012, Revision 2–May 2012, Revision 3–July 2022). Retrieved from https://mutcd.fhwa.dot.gov/

U.S. Fire Administration. (2012). *Traffic Incident Management Systems*. Report FA-330. Retrieved from https://www.usfa.fema.gov/downloads/pdf/publications/fa_330.pdf

# REFERENCES

Bullough, J. D., Parr, S. A., Sbledorio, A., & Hiebner, E. (2021). *Effects of emergency vehicle lighting characteristics on driver perception and behavior*. Emergency Responder Institute. Retrieved from https://www.respondersafety.com/Download.aspx?DownloadId=f31a5f73-7b95-44c7-bd25-1e4cdfce5229

Centers for Disease Control and Prevention. (2003). Ambulance crash-related injuries among emergency medical services workers—United States, 1991–2002. *Morbidity and Mortality Weekly Report, 52*(8), 154–156. Retrieved from http://www.cdc.gov/mmwr/preview/mmwrhtml/mm5208a3.htm

Centers for Disease Control and Prevention. (2011, January). *Policy impact: Seat belts*. Retrieved from https://www.cdc.gov/transportationsafety/seatbeltbrief/index.html

Centers for Disease Control and Prevention. (2022, November). *Drowsy driving: Asleep at the wheel*. Retrieved from https://www.cdc.gov/sleep/features/drowsy-driving.html

Emergency Responder Safety Institute. (2022). *2022 emergency responder struck-by-vehicle fatalities*. Retrieved from https://www.respondersafety.com/Download.aspx?DownloadId=1daeaf45-d126-4ff5-8f8e-2392f1af7f3f

McCallion, T. (2012). Consider the dangers of shift work: It's important to have a fatigue management plan in place. *Journal of Emergency Medical Services*. Retrieved from http://www.jems.com/article/emsinsider/consider-dangers-shift-work

National Highway Traffic Safety Administration. Fatality Analysis Reporting System (FARS) 2013 Annual Report File (ARF).

National Institute for Occupational Safety and Health. (2004). *Emergency medical technician dies in ambulance crash—New York*. Fatality Assessment and Control Evaluation (FACE) Program. Retrieved from http://www.cdc.gov/niosh/face/In-house/full200112.html

National Sleep Foundation. (n.d.). Drowsy driving: Too tired to drive. Retrieved from https://www.thensf.org/ddpw-tf/

National Sleep Foundation. (2022, November 2). *New data from the National Sleep Foundation show a majority of Americans drive while drowsy*. Retrieved from https://www.thensf.org/new-data-from-the-national-sleep-foundation-show-a-majority-of-americans-drive-while-drowsy/

National Sleep Foundation. (2022). Sleep first. Drive alert. Retrieved from https://www.thensf.org/drowsy-driving-prevention/

U.S. Department of Transportation, Federal Highway Administration. (2020). *Traffic incident management quick clearance laws: A national review of best practices*. Retrieved from https://ops.fhwa.dot.gov/publications/fhwahop09005/move_over.htm

# CHAPTER 3

# EMS Vehicle Operation and the Law

## OBJECTIVES

**3.1** Define the types of laws that affect EMS vehicle operation.

**3.2** Explain the legal terms related to EMS vehicle operation.

**3.3** Explain why it is important to know your state's laws pertinent to emergency vehicle operations.

**3.4** Describe the appropriate use of lights and siren.

**3.5** Discuss safety considerations for responding to an emergency scene.

**3.6** Outline the types of preventable collisions most common to emergency vehicle operations.

**3.7** Discuss the assessment of liability and how liability affects the emergency vehicle operator.

**3.8** Explain steps the emergency vehicle operator can take to avoid legal entanglements.

**3.9** Describe how to respond appropriately in the event of a collision.

## SCENARIO

You and your partner are at the daily meeting in the center of town when a Priority 1 response is dispatched for your zone. As you drive past the airport, with your lights and siren on, you approach a red traffic light. There is no traffic to the left and a few vehicles to your right. Though they have a green light, they are stopped at the intersection. You slow down slightly and proceed through the intersection. Suddenly, almost out of nowhere, a BMW pulls directly in front of your ambulance from the right. You react quickly and hit the brakes, but your vehicle still hits the driver's side door.

You are unharmed. You quickly check on your partner; he says he is okay but that his sternum is sore. Next, you get out to check on the driver of the other vehicle. She is conscious, alert, and oriented, and still in the driver's seat. Her left leg appears to be broken. She also appears to be trapped in the vehicle and will require extrication.

*(continues)*

## INTRODUCTION

This chapter introduces the legal considerations for emergency vehicle operators (EVOs). Service policy makers and their driver trainers should outline very clearly what your responsibilities are for operating the emergency vehicle. They should also provide high-quality training to you to prepare you for your job. Department leadership should also remain current with all laws and policies that pertain to driving emergency vehicles in your jurisdiction. However, it is ultimately *your* responsibility to properly perform your job and know the laws that govern your actions. If you are involved in a crash in which someone is seriously injured or killed and you broke traffic laws, violated department SOPs, or acted without due regard to others (a subject discussed later), you could face legal consequences, possibly even manslaughter or negligent homicide charges in the case of a fatality.

### SAFETY TIP

The EVO should be familiar with the state traffic laws, specific municipality ordinances, and all department SOPs related to emergency vehicle operation. This can also include mutual aid and neighboring communities that you travel through.

# Criminal and Civil Law

The U.S. judicial system is divided into two primary types of law, criminal and civil. **Criminal law** involves determining whether a statute has been violated and, if so, assessing an appropriate punishment, whether that is a fine, jail or prison incarceration, or both. For a minor criminal offense, such as illegally parking your ambulance when not on an emergency call, a police officer could issue a citation requiring you to appear in front of a judge, who would most likely impose a fine. For a more serious criminal offense, such as striking and killing a pedestrian, the vehicle operator could be arrested and placed in jail and would need to arrange for legal representation in the ensuing criminal proceedings.

Motor vehicle laws involve the criminal justice system. If you violate a traffic law, such as exceeding the speed limit in your personal vehicle, you have committed a criminal offense. While emergency vehicles are given a certain amount of latitude with regard to following motor vehicle laws, emergency vehicle operators may still be ticketed or fined if they disregard these laws and put the public at risk.

**Civil law** is much broader and more often invoked against a vehicle operator in cases of vehicle collisions (even when the incident does not lead to criminal charges). In a civil action, an injured person files a lawsuit naming the vehicle operator as the **defendant**. The **plaintiff** (person suing) asks for monetary compensation for their physical, emotional, and psychological injuries as well as other damages, such as loss of employability or other financial harm.

In criminal cases, the state (or prosecution) must prove to a jury that the accused is guilty of the crime beyond a **reasonable doubt**, meaning that a reasonable person would not doubt the accused party's guilt. In civil cases, however, the plaintiff must prove their case based on only a **preponderance of the evidence**, meaning there is slightly more evidence of guilt than of innocence. In a civil case, the jury may choose to award the plaintiff compensation from the defendant at the requested amount or at a higher or lower amount, based on the jury's determination of the defendant's level of guilt.

# Legal Terms

The most common cause of legal trouble for a vehicle operator is a collision. In a vehicle collision, there may be criminal charges brought against the operator, but much more likely there will be a civil suit naming the operator as a defendant. In civil suits involving collisions, the primary goal is to establish **liability**, which is the determination of who is primarily at fault for the collision. In civil cases involving emergency vehicles, the primary determination of liability is based on a term called **negligence**, which indicates that the vehicle operator did not perform their responsibilities correctly. To prove negligence in a vehicle collision, the plaintiff must prove that the defendant had a responsibility to act in a certain way and that they failed to do so, resulting in a collision that caused injury to the plaintiff.

**Gross negligence** is a more serious form of negligence, and implies reckless conduct and a blatant disregard for the safety and lives of others. Consider, for example, a vehicle operator driving under the influence of alcohol who collides with a vehicle that is stopped at an intersection and kills the vehicle's driver upon impact. To prove gross negligence, the plaintiff would need to prove that the defendant's conduct was deliberately reckless and without concern for other drivers' safety. The line between negligence and gross negligence can be unclear and may need to be determined by a court.

In the event of a collision involving an emergency medical services (EMS) vehicle, a court primarily bases its judgment on these two questions:

1. Did the emergency vehicle operator have reasonable grounds to believe they were responding to a *true emergency*?
2. Did the emergency vehicle operator exercise *due regard* for the safety of others?

---

## OPERATOR INCIDENT

The following comparisons are based on incidents that can tragically occur somewhere almost every day. Note how differently the incident appears to the public when it involves an ambulance.

In a suburban neighborhood, there was a tragic crash that involved a preschool-aged child on a "big wheel," who rolled down his driveway and entered the street. A pine tree at the foot of the driveway was a potential obstruction to the view of the oncoming traffic. Two middle-aged couples were in a car traveling through this suburban neighborhood on their way to dinner. They were traveling at the posted speed limit. The child suddenly darted out in front of them, and they did not see the child before striking and fatally injuring him. While EMS was attempting to resuscitate the child, police took statements from witnesses, did a field sobriety test, and checked for skid marks as a part of their investigation. The child was promptly transported to the trauma center and did not survive. In the end, there was no traffic ticket issued because it was determined that the driver of the vehicle could not have avoided hitting the child.

In another collision a few months later in a different community, an ambulance was responding with lights and siren to a call on a residential street. They were exceeding the posted speed limit but not by more than the 10 mph that their department SOP allowed. A school-aged child rode his bicycle into the side of the ambulance. He was not wearing a helmet and he sustained a fatal head injury. The EMS crew heard a loud noise and noticed the cyclist had smashed into the side of the ambulance. They immediately stopped and called for police, their supervisor, and for the initial call to be reassigned. They tried to revive the child, a second ambulance crew arrived and promptly transported him to the trauma center, yet the child did not survive. The police again interviewed witnesses, measured skid marks, and did a field sobriety test of the EVO. In this case, although no evidence appeared to indicate that the EMS crew was at fault and no tickets were issued, the case was turned over to the grand jury for further investigation. The media attacked the EMS service and published the name and address of the EVO. Weeks later, the grand jury determined that the crash could not have been avoided and the EVO was not at fault, but the service's and operator's reputations were deeply damaged.

As you can see from these two similar cases, the due regard provision sets a higher standard for EVOs. Always make every effort to take due regard for the safety of others while operating an EMS vehicle.

A **true emergency** is a situation in which there is a high probability of death or serious injury to an individual or of significant property loss, and the actions of the responders can mitigate the situation. **Due regard** refers to taking appropriate considerations in a given situation. The determination of "appropriate" is based on what a reasonably careful person could be expected to do if they were performing similar duties under similar circumstances. Thus, "due regard for the safety of others" means taking precautions that a reasonably prudent person would take to safeguard the public in a similar situation.

The law gives a tremendous amount of responsibility to EVOs when a call is classified as a true emergency; however, operators must still show due regard for the safety of all others. To show due regard, the EVO must give sufficient notice of the vehicle's approach (e.g., lights and siren) to allow other motorists and pedestrians to clear a path and protect themselves. If you do not give notice of your approach until a collision is unavoidable, you have not satisfied the principle of due regard for the safety of others.

### SAFETY TIP

The emergency vehicle operator (EVO) is held to a higher standard than all other drivers on the road.

# Know Your State's Requirements

In a 2019 survey of state EMS offices, the following highlights were noted:

- Definition of ambulance: 92% of states have official definitions of an ambulance. While definitions differed in length and content, all included a provision that to be an ambulance, the vehicle must be designed for the transport of a sick or injured person to a medical facility.
- Regulation of ambulance agencies: All reported state-level regulation or oversight of ambulance provider agencies. While names of the state agencies varied, most regulation of ambulance providers fell under the equivalent of a state Department of Health (81.5%) or a separate EMS Authority/Regulatory Board (13.2%). A few states (5.3%) reported oversight from state Department of Public Safety or its equivalent. Licensing or permitting of local EMS agencies was the most common type of regulation and oversight provided by state EMS offices.

- Agencies authorized to operate ambulances: Most states could provide counts of the number of EMS agencies that were licensed, and many did not differentiate between volunteer and professional agencies in their counts because the regulations and licensure requirements for these EMS provider agencies are the same in most instances.
- Regulation of ambulance operators/drivers: Most states acknowledged that few agencies have staff members whose only function is to drive ambulances. The majority (84.2%) of states reported that the same department providing regulation and oversight for ambulance agencies also regulated individual ambulance operators. Four states reported that individual ambulance operators were not regulated at the state level. One state said its Department of Motor Vehicles (DMV) oversaw ambulance operators, and one state reported operator regulation by the state Fire Prevention Commission. In California, the ambulance driver certificate (which differs from a standard driver's license) is issued by the state after passing a written exam, paying a fee, fingerprinting, and a medical report. No other state had a state-run test (written or on road) of operators other than a standard driver's license. Only six states reported checking the driving history of ambulance operators before they could operate an ambulance. In those states, common disqualifying events included impaired driving, reckless driving, and a license suspension due to drugs/alcohol or a severe moving violation.
- Emergency vehicle operator course (EVOC) requirements: 17 states had specific requirements that an ambulance operator complete an EVOC, but most did not keep records of who had completed the course. In most cases, the local EMS agency was responsible for ensuring the EVOC was completed when required by the state. Only two states reported having any control over who was qualified to teach the ambulance EVOC. Nine states had lists of approved EVOCs, but only five of them had some form of minimum requirements for the topics that must be covered. Only five states specifically required behind-the-wheel components to the training.
- Refresher/remedial operator training: Seven states required refresher training for operators. When required, it generally took place every 1 to 3 years and was of shorter duration than a full EVOC. No states required remedial EVOC training after a crash.
- Evaluation: No states reported conducting a formal evaluation of the effectiveness of an EVOC.

# Use of Lights and Siren

Lights and siren (L&S) are used to alert motorists and pedestrians of the approach of an emergency vehicle. State laws mandate that the EVO use emergency warning devices such as L&S when reasonably necessary, especially when taking advantage of any traffic law exemptions (**Figure 3-1**). However, the use of signaling equipment does not guarantee that motorists and pedestrians will be aware of the presence of the vehicle, nor do they protect the vehicle operator from civil or criminal liability if a collision occurs.

States require the use of both lights and siren. The use of lights only is actually more of a hazard since other motorists do not understand what the situation is. Simply transporting a patient does not constitute the use of lights; if the patient's clinical condition is stable and the vehicle is obeying the vehicle and traffic laws (VTL) without exemption, there is no need for the lights to be activated. If the patient is unstable and their clinical condition requires expedited transport, then both lights and siren (L&S) are to be used. (This requirement is subject to laws, rule, regulations, and agency SOP.) The siren needs to be on continually so that traffic beyond the immediate vicinity is alerted; simply "chirping" the siren when approaching intersections does not provide adequate notice to other motorists and can actually startle drivers who aren't immediately able to locate the emergency vehicle. (Note that this is required for fire and EMS responses; however, in many jurisdictions, law enforcement is exempt, due in part to their need to arrive silently on certain sensitive calls.)

Legally, your emergency warning devices require traffic to yield the right of way. However, you have no guarantee that you will receive the right of way. Motorists or pedestrians who do not give you the right of way

may be breaking the law, but you are still required to give them due regard.

The use of emergency lights must comply with state and local laws, state and local EMS rules and regulations, and your department's SOPs. In addition, the Joint Statement on Lights & Siren Vehicle Operations on EMS Responses (Chapter 1) may be cited in legal proceedings involving L&S use.

For the reasons already stated, the lights do not provide as much protection or warning as you may think. Furthermore, some believe that when parking at the scene of an emergency, the use of the warning lights could actually make the scene unsafe by reducing the visibility of other drivers beyond the flashing lights, especially during low light conditions. Flashing lights may also draw the driver's eye, distracting their attention from the road. It is important to remember that low sun, glare, fog, and tinted windows in other vehicles can reduce the effectiveness of warning lights.

At night, red warning lights may blend in with other red lights in traffic or the neon lights along the side of the streets. Warning lights mounted on top of a vehicle may not be visible in the rearview mirror of vehicles in front of the emergency vehicle.

There are similar concerns with the effectiveness of the siren. In general, a siren can be heard only to a distance of 230 feet ahead of the vehicle. At speeds greater than 40 mph, you can completely outpace the effectiveness of your siren. Even at close range, the siren may not be heard by a motorist who has the vehicle's windows closed and is using the air conditioning or radio. Newer cars even advertise how much outside noise the car's insulation blocks, and this includes an emergency vehicle's siren.

## Lights and Siren: What About the Patient in Out-of-Hospital Cardiac Arrest?

The best response to a confirmed out-of-hospital cardiac arrest (OHCA) is careful use of L&S by the first arriving unit, with a clear report to additional units responding to downgrade their response if appropriate. Remember the fastest response is "zero response" by utilizing dispatcher-assisted cardiopulmonary resuscitation (DA-CPR), training bystanders, placing automated external defibrillators (AEDs) in public locations, and a safe response.

Once at the scene, either initiate resuscitation measures and achieve return of spontaneous circulation (ROSC) or exhaust on-scene protocols and call for a physician termination order (in accordance with agency medical direction and local/regional/state protocols). Remember the greatest chance of successful ROSC involves

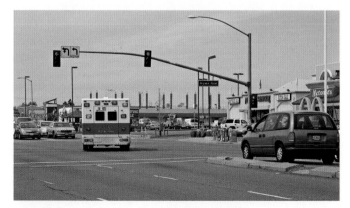

**Figure 3-1** Emergency warning devices should be used when taking any exemptions to vehicle and traffic laws.
© Karin Hildebrand Lau/Alamy Stock Photo

DA-CPR, bystander CPR, and AED as soon as possible. In most communities, ambulances do not transport the deceased, certainly not with L&S.

If you are transporting an OHCA patient, that means one of the following occurred:

- You obtained ROSC, so the patient needs to be carefully managed and taken to a cardiac arrest center.
- The patient coded in the back of the ambulance and after an appropriate response (the EVO pulls the ambulance over to safe location, calls for additional assistance, and assists the crew in managing the OHCA), a mechanical compression device is applied or ROSC is attained and the EVO resumes safe transport to appropriate facility.
- The patient was a critical trauma patient who lost their pulse and is being resuscitated in the ambulance while slowly and carefully proceeding to the most appropriate facility.

**SAFETY TIP**

Remember that the fastest response is "zero response," in which initial care is provided by bystanders prior to EMS arrival. This is achieved by utilizing dispatcher-assisted cardiopulmonary resuscitation (DA-CPR), training community members in CPR, and placing automated external defibrillators (AEDs) in public locations.

# Responding Safely

When responding to an incident, EVOs should be told if they are being dispatched on a potential emergency. Dispatch should obtain information from the caller to determine how the EVO should respond (i.e., emergency or nonemergency) by using an emergency medical dispatch system. EMS system directors may be liable if they do not have a policy regarding what information responders should receive when they are dispatched.

Nonemergency responses include incidents involving chronic illness (without life-threatening complications), minor injuries, and stable patients. True emergencies include cardiac or respiratory complications, major trauma, or other life-threatening complaints based on your system's 911 dispatch categories. In EMS systems, the EVO should initiate a high-priority response to a presumed, true emergency that includes the use of emergency warning devices. The response mode may change or downgrade if a first responder, on the scene, is reporting that the call does not involve a life-threatening situation.

The decision about routine or emergency transport, from the scene to the emergency department, should be made by asking the following questions:

- Will the time saved make a significant difference in the patient's outcome?
- Will emergency transport create an unnecessarily unsafe situation for the public, myself and my partner(s), and the patient?
- What effect will the emergency warning devices have on the surrounding public, patient, driver, and crew?

It is important to note that in situations in which it is necessary to respond to the station or emergency scene in your own private vehicle, you must adhere to all applicable motor vehicle laws. Privately owned nonemergency vehicles are not granted any exemptions or special privileges by most states and must obey all state vehicle and traffic laws, even when states allow the use of emergency warning devices. State rules and department SOPs vary greatly in what they consider an authorized emergency vehicle. Regardless, if you are responding in a nonemergency vehicle, you should make a special effort to drive in a safe manner. As with emergency vehicles, you should pay close attention to speed limits, road and weather conditions, intersections, and maneuvering your vehicle around the emergency scene.

If your private vehicle has an emergency identification light, you must comply with the applicable emergency motor vehicle rules and regulations that cover size, type, color, and candle power of the light. You must also recognize that you are representing your emergency response organization and drawing attention to yourself when you respond with a light on your private vehicle. You might consider shutting off the light when you are stopped at traffic lights or stop signs to avoid distracting motorists and pedestrians (**Figure 3-2**). Always follow the

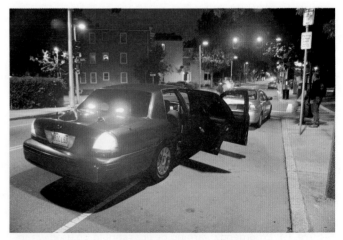

**Figure 3-2** Private vehicles may be issued emergency warning devices for emergency response.
© Michael Matthews - Police Images/Alamy Stock Photo

SOPs of your department and any state laws concerning the use of colored lights on personal vehicles.

<br>

**SAFETY TIP**

You can be held both criminally and civilly liable if a collision occurs while you are on duty as an emergency responder. The agency for which you work can also be brought into a lawsuit if the case can be made that you were improperly or inadequately instructed or that no effort was made to control unsafe or reckless vehicle operation.

## Is There Still a "Golden Hour"?

The idea of the "golden hour" in trauma, in which seriously injured patients who arrive at definitive care within 60 minutes of injury have the best outcomes, has been a part of emergency care since its conception in the 1960s. While this theory seems reasonable (many injuries cannot be completely controlled in the field and require surgical intervention or in-hospital treatment), the research does not conclusively support it.

In a study of more than 3,000 trauma patients presenting with hypotension, head injury, or difficulty breathing, researchers compared response times (both total times and time in each phase of response) to patient outcomes and determined that shorter intervals did not result in improved survival rates, at least in patients with circulatory, respiratory, or neurologic impairment. Other studies report similar findings.

This is not to suggest that responses times are irrelevant; rapid transport to definitive care is critical for many trauma patients. What the research does show, however, is that time is *not* the most important component of EMS response, and that focusing on meeting a specific time limit may result in suboptimal patient care. This is an especially important consideration when designing quality control guidelines, as response time is a common benchmark used in EMS systems.

With all of this in mind, many systems and EMS curricula have moved toward the idea of the "golden period," which retains the importance of rapid response without overly focusing on a specific time frame. Current research suggests that the amount of time spent on scene is more important to patient outcomes than transport time. For a critical trauma patient, limiting on-scene time by performing a rapid assessment, initiating only those interventions necessary to correct life threats, and promptly packaging the patient for transport to the appropriate facility produce better outcomes than speeding or otherwise trying to save time on the transport itself. Driving faster does little more than putting everyone on the road, as well as your crew, your patient, and yourself, at risk.

## Types of Collisions

One of the most common causes of legal issues for an EVO is a collision involving the emergency vehicle they are driving. There are many types of collisions common to emergency vehicle operations. The ones most likely to involve legal trouble for the operator are preventable collisions.

A **preventable collision** is one in which the driver failed to do everything reasonable to prevent its occurrence. Note that the word *reasonable*, rather than *possible*, is used in this definition; there is always something possible that could have been done to prevent a collision (such as not responding to the call or taking another street). Reasonable preventive measures include knowing, understanding, and obeying traffic laws; adjusting speed to existing conditions; scanning ahead to anticipate stops; and anticipating the reactions of other drivers and pedestrians to your emergency vehicle.

There are many different types of preventable collisions:

- Parking collisions may result from double-parking, failure to warn traffic of your parked position, and parking in an unconventional location, to name a few examples.
- Intersection collisions are those that happen at stop lights, stop signs, or other intersections, where different directions of traffic must cross paths.
- Backing collisions occur while the vehicle is in reverse gear.
- In rear-end collisions, the emergency vehicle impacts a vehicle in front of it; these incidents are commonly caused by not maintaining a safe following distance, not looking ahead to anticipate the need to stop, or not controlling vehicle speed.
- Pedestrian collisions are always considered preventable, even though children and adults may perform sudden, unexpected maneuvers.
- Mechanical failure collisions are often the result of lack of attention during the vehicle inspection, reckless or abusive vehicle handling, or operating the vehicle beyond its mechanical limits (e.g., over the gross vehicle weight rating).
- Adverse weather collisions may be caused by failure to drive according to the existing conditions, failure to postpone nonemergency calls, failure to use snow chains, or driving in adverse weather conditions.
- Traffic lane encroachment collisions may be the result of using improper passing techniques, weaving through or merging with traffic at unsafe times, or changing lanes in an unsafe manner.
- Collisions with fixed objects such as low overheads, buildings, poles, parked cars, and trees, or collisions

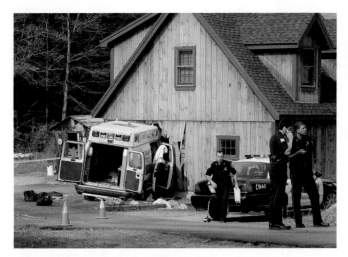

**Figure 3-3** Collisions into stationary objects are considered preventable collisions.

© Jon Hill/The Lowell Sun/AP Photo

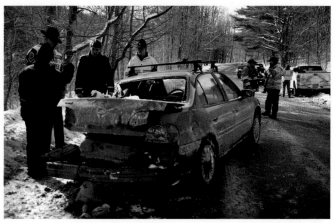

**Figure 3-4** Always cooperate with a crash scene investigation.

© Valley News, photographer: Jennifer Hauck

resulting from running off the roadway or overturning the vehicle may be caused by unsafe evasive action on the part of the emergency vehicle operator (**Figure 3-3**).

# Criminal and Civil Law

## Liability in Cases of Collisions

As mentioned earlier, liability is the determination of who is primarily at fault in the event of a collision. In addition to evaluating whether the emergency vehicle was responding to a true emergency with due regard for the safety of others, the judge or jury may ask the following questions:

- Are there any state, national, or department standards for emergency vehicle operation that may apply? If so, did the specific EVO comply with them?
- Do any state statutes regarding emergency vehicle exemptions apply?
- Was the EVO properly trained and supervised per accepted standards, and did the operator follow the SOPs of the agency?
- Was the vehicle properly equipped, was the equipment being properly operated, and are there records of relevant repairs and preventive maintenance?
- Were the manufacturer's ratings exceeded?
- Did the emergency vehicle have seatbelts, and if so, were they properly utilized?

A finding of liability in a vehicle collision involving an ambulance will likely result in monetary damages being assessed to the vehicle operator, as well as the EMS

service they represent. It is in everyone's best interest for the EVO to avoid any action that might result in a collision for which they might be liable.

# Avoiding Legal Entanglements

Ultimately, it is the EVO's responsibility to know and obey the laws of your state and the SOPs of your organization as they relate to driving an emergency vehicle. State laws may vary regarding the maximum speed at which emergency vehicles can drive during an emergency operation and which traffic law exemptions emergency vehicles have, but in all states, emergency vehicle operators must drive with due regard for the safety of others. The best way to stay out of legal entanglements is to be attentive and practice safe driving.

If you do become involved in a collision, stay calm, follow your agency's SOP, and notify the police. Care for any injured persons immediately and always remain courteous and polite. You should not make any statements to the media but should cooperate with any investigations or police documentation (**Figure 3-4**).

New laws relevant to emergency services are enacted every year, and while not all rules and regulations are directly related to emergency vehicle operations, it is critical that the EVO remain up to date regarding these changes. For example, multiple states have enacted a law that makes it a crime for first responders (EMS, fire, and law enforcement personnel) to share images or video from motor vehicle crashes publicly, including posting on social media, without the consent of the parties involved. In some states, the law also allows victims to bring civil suits against the individuals and agencies involved, which could result in the awarding of monetary awards to the victims as well as irreparable damage to the agency's public image.

Many fire and EMS departments currently have SOPs that limit or prevent the use of personal phones and cameras at emergency scenes. What is your agency's policy?

## CRASH ANALYSIS

### Fatal Rural 911 Response in Ohio

This crash involved a 2017 Ford Transit Type II ambulance and a 2014 Dodge Ram 2500 truck and occurred on a rural two-lane roadway. It was evening dusk (twilight) conditions without any artificial lighting, 50°F with moderate rainfall. The posted speed limit was 55 mph and analysis of the event data recorder (EDR) reported speed revealed the ambulance was traveling 62 mph and the Dodge truck was traveling at 51 mph moments before the crash. Aside from the Dodge truck's loss of control, reports noted insufficient tire tread for the wet road conditions. The crash resulted in the death of the ambulance's unbelted 43-year-old female paramedic who was sitting in the front right passenger seat. At the time of the crash, the ambulance was responding to a medical emergency (unconscious patient) in a nursing home approximately 10 miles from the ambulance's point of dispatch. The warning lights and siren were in use. It was driven by a belted 28-year-old male EMT. The

Dodge truck lost control and crossed over the roadway's centerline into the path of the ambulance. Following the crash, both occupants were transported by other ambulances to local hospitals for treatment. The female passenger was pronounced dead within hours of the crash, while the driver sustained incapacitating but nonlife-threatening injuries. The driver of the Dodge truck also suffered serious but nonlife-threatening injuries.

The private ambulance service has a policy of initial and ongoing EVO training as well as an aggressive fatigue prevention SOP.

1. What were some of the contributing factors to this tragic crash?
2. Realizing that not all nursing homes and their staff are the same, is it worth the risk of a L&S response to an unconscious patient in a "medical facility" under the care of "medical providers"?

Modified from Crash Research & Analysis. *Special Crash Investigations: On-Site Ambulance Crash Investigation; Vehicle: 2017 Ford Transit Type II Ambulance; Location; Ohio; Crash date: October 2018* (Report No. DOT HS 813 257). National Highway Traffic Safety Administration. February 2022. https://crashstats.nhtsa.dot.gov/Api/Public/ViewPublication/813257

## SUMMARY

- Criminal law involves determining whether a statute has been violated and, if so, assessing an appropriate punishment, whether that be a fine, jail or prison incarceration, or both.

- Civil law is much broader and more often invoked against a vehicle operator in cases of vehicle collisions (even when the incident does not lead to criminal charges).

- In criminal cases, the state (or prosecution) must prove to a jury that the accused is guilty of the crime beyond a reasonable doubt, meaning that a reasonable person would not doubt the accused party's guilt.

- In civil cases, the plaintiff must prove their case based on only a preponderance of the evidence, meaning there is slightly more evidence of guilt than of innocence.

- A true emergency is a situation in which there is a high probability of death or serious injury to an individual or of significant property loss, and the actions of the responders can mitigate the situation.

- Due regard is taking appropriate considerations in a given situation. The determination of "appropriate" is based on what a reasonably careful person could be expected to do if they were performing similar duties under similar circumstances.

- Lights and siren are used to alert motorists and pedestrians of the approach of an emergency vehicle. State laws mandate that the EVO use emergency warning devices such as lights and/or siren when reasonably necessary, especially when taking advantage of any traffic law exemptions.

- A preventable collision is one in which the driver failed to do everything reasonable to prevent its occurrence. Note that the word *reasonable*, rather than *possible*, is used in this definition.

- The best way to stay out of legal entanglements is to be attentive and practice safe driving.

## GLOSSARY

**civil law** The type of law that pertains to determining responsibility for a wrongful act and imposing monetary penalties (with or without criminal charges) if the defendant is found guilty.

**criminal law** The type of law that pertains to determining whether a statute has been violated and, if so, imposing a punishment (fine and/or imprisonment) on the guilty party.

**defendant** The person or party in a lawsuit who is charged with breaking the law and harming the plaintiff.

**due regard** Appropriate consideration and responsibility shown for the safety of others.

**gross negligence** A more serious form of negligence that implies reckless conduct and a blatant disregard for the safety and lives of others. The line between negligence and gross negligence may need to be determined by a court.

**liability** Legal accountability or obligation.

**negligence** Failure to exercise due caution.

**plaintiff** The person or party who files a complaint in a lawsuit claiming to have been harmed by the defendant.

**preponderance of the evidence** A requirement in determining the guilt of a defendant that the majority of evidence presented in a case favor the plaintiff's argument.

**preventable collision** A collision in which the driver failed to do everything reasonable to prevent its occurrence.

**reasonable doubt** The lack of certainty that a person may justifiably feel based on the evidence at hand regarding the alleged guilt of a defendant.

**true emergency** A situation in which there is a high probability of death or serious injury to an individual or of significant property loss.

## REFERENCES

Crash Research & Analysis, Inc. (2022, February). Special Crash Investigations: *On-site ambulance crash investigation; Vehicle: 2017 Ford Transit Type II Ambulance;* Location; Ohio; Crash date: October 2018 (Report No. DOT HS 813 257). NHTSA.

DeLorenzo, P. A., & Eilers, M. A. (1995). Lights and siren: A review of emergency vehicle warning systems. *Annals of Emergency Medicine, 20*(12), 1331–1335.

Meisel, Z., & Pines, J. (2010). High-speed care: How fast should ambulances go? *Slate.* Retrieved from https://slate.com/technology/2010/05/how-fast-should-ambulances-go.html

National Association of Emergency Medical Technicians. (2023). *Prehospital Trauma Life Support* (10th ed.). Burlington, MA: Jones and Bartlett Learning.

Newgard, C. D., Schmicker, R. H., Hedges, J. Ry., et al., & Resuscitation Outcomes Consortium Investigators. (2010). Emergency medical services intervals and survival in trauma: Assessment of the golden hour in a North American prospective cohort. *Annals of Emergency Medicine, 55*(3), 235–246.

Nikolaou, N., Dainty, K. N., Couper, K., Morley, P., Tijssen, J., Vaillancourt, C.; on behalf of the International Liaison Committee on Resuscitation's (ILCOR) Basic Life Support and Pediatric Task Forces. (2019). A systematic review and meta-analysis of the effect of dispatcher-assisted CPR on outcomes from sudden cardiac arrest in adults and children. *Resuscitation, 138,* 82–105. doi: 10.1016/j.resuscitation.2019.02.035

Panchal, A. R., Berg, K. M., Cabañas, J. G., Kurz, M. C., Link, M.S., Del Rios, M., et al. (2019). 2019 American Heart Association focused update on systems of care: Dispatcher-assisted cardiopulmonary resuscitation and cardiac arrest centers: An update to the American Heart Association Guidelines for Cardiopulmonary Resuscitation and Emergency Cardiovascular Care. *Circulation, 140,* e895–e903. doi: 10.1161/CIR.0000000000000733

Thomas, F. D., Graham, L. A., Wright, T. J., Almedia, R., Blomberg, R. D., & Benlemlih, M. (2019, December). *Characterizing ambulance driver training in EMS systems* (Report No. DOT HS 812 862). National Highway Traffic Safety Administration.

Zoller, B. P. (n.d.). New state laws address photographs of victims by first responders. *XpertHR.* Retrieved from https://www.xperthr.com/news/new-state-laws-address-photographs-of-victims-by-first-responders/7692/

# CHAPTER 4

# Vehicle Inspection and Maintenance

## OBJECTIVES

**4.1** Explain the importance of vehicle inspection and preventive maintenance.

**4.2** Demonstrate how to perform a complete vehicle inspection of the exterior and interior.

**4.3** Explain the function, inspection, and maintenance procedures for the various mechanical components and systems of your emergency vehicle.

**4.4** Explain how to respond appropriately to vehicle problems.

**4.5** Discuss the value of road testing for vehicle performance.

**4.6** Describe relevant standards and certification programs for vehicle inspection and maintenance.

## SCENARIO

Kelsey moved the ambulance out of the bay for the morning checkout and noticed a pool of fluid on the bay floor. She noted the presence of fluid on her checkout sheet and reported the problem to her supervisor. The supervisor asked what color the fluid was, but Kelsey did not know. She returned to the bay area to look, but someone had already mopped the bay and cleaned up the fluid.

The supervisor explained that color is an important clue to determine what type of fluid is leaking. For example, motor oil is typically golden to black in color, antifreeze is typically green and watery, and transmission fluid is red with an oil-like consistency. By noting the color of the fluid, Kelsey would have been able to make an educated guess about potential vehicle problems.

1. Do you have a clear list of reasons for when and how an ambulance can be marked out for mechanical problems?
2. What are your standard operating procedures (SOPs) and training for checking the mechanical elements of the ambulance?
3. As an operator, what liability do you hold for the mechanical function of the ambulance?

## INTRODUCTION

As the emergency vehicle operator (EVO), you are responsible for the proper mechanical operation of your vehicle. This does not mean that you need to be a mechanic, but you should have at least enough understanding of how the vehicle operates to identify potential problems before they occur. It is also important to understand your role and responsibility based on your department's policy. Each department will have different standards for which the EVO will be responsible.

# Vehicle Inspection

Most emergency services require daily inspections of vehicles and equipment. Daily checks can help manage any known or developing problems with the vehicle by identifying trends as well as finding anything unexpected. Most services have a mandatory checklist that is completed on a routine basis (**Figure 4-1**). Never complete a vehicle inspection checklist without verifying each element on it. You should complete a thorough inspection of the entire vehicle prior to each shift to ensure there is no damage to the vehicle or any safety hazards that could affect the vehicle's performance. This inspection includes the vehicle's exterior, the interior compartments, and the functional systems and mechanical components. As the operator of an emergency vehicle, it is your responsibility to be aware of the function, conduct an inspection, and perform basic maintenance of the various components of the vehicle for which you are responsible. This chapter provides a general introduction to vehicle maintenance assuming a standard ambulance; EVOs who operate more specialized vehicles should receive more specific training.

> **SAFETY TIP**
>
> During the vehicle inspection, emergency personnel should review the location and confirm the presence of all emergency equipment. Vehicle inspection checklists are legal documents that can be subpoenaed, so take your documentation seriously.

## Exterior Inspection

All services want to present a professional appearance, and many people base opinions about a service simply on the appearance of the vehicle. Therefore, during the inspection, you should check that the vehicle body is clean and free of damage, noting any new damage that may not have been reported. Next, examine the tires to ensure they are in good condition and have adequate tread, with no bulges along the sidewall. Any uneven wear should be noted, and the spare tire (if present) should also be examined. The air pressure in the tires should be checked to make sure they are properly inflated. Remember that the proper inflation is determined by the vehicle manufacturer and not the tire manufacturer. Variations in tire inflation, such as a reduction of 3–4 psi (10%) can alter handling, fuel economy, and braking distance.

All external lights should be checked for proper operation, including emergency lights in responding and traffic-blocking modes. Check for signs of internal moisture and for rusted reflectors inside the lights, and also make sure the lights are securely fastened. To safely check emergency lights in the responding mode, it is necessary for the engine to be running with the transmission in park and the parking brake activated. This will activate the high idle, which supports the power drain of the emergency lights. (Newer vehicles with light-emitting diode (LED) lighting will not have the same power drain as incandescent lighting.) Next, put the transmission into drive with the parking brake engaged, and while one person has a foot on the brake, have another person walk around the vehicle to check for proper operation of each light, including turn signals. By completing a 360-degree walk around the vehicle to check the lighting, you also have the perspective of other drivers on the road that will see your vehicle. Not having lighting that works properly will hinder other drivers from being able to see you.

Newer vehicles may have both response and scene mode lighting. When the vehicle is in drive, all emergency lighting will engage, and when the vehicle is in park, most of the flashing lights on various parts of the vehicle will shut down, and some vehicles will reduce the intensity of the remaining lights. If you vehicle supports more than one lighting mode, ensure that all modes activate correctly.

While testing the emergency lights, the EVO should briefly test the siren to ensure that it sounds properly when needed. Use caution when testing the siren due to high noise levels it creates. It is helpful to test the siren with bay doors open (or outdoors). Also, ensure that no one is standing in front of the vehicle while testing the siren.

Once the walk-around is complete, turn off all emergency lights, put the vehicle in park, and turn the engine off. Check that all doors open, close, and lock properly, including door locks on the patient compartment. Examine the windows; they should be clean and free of cracks and should open properly if designed to do so. The external antennas should be intact and secure. The exhaust system should be intact and directed toward the side or rear of the vehicle, as appropriate. The windshield should be clean and free of cracks and debris. The windshield wipers should include pliable wiping material that cleans the windshield without leaving any streaks. Dry and cracked wipers need to be replaced. To check the windshield washer level, look at the reservoir inside the engine compartment. If the level appears low, add washer fluid to fill the reservoir according to company policy.

## Daily Ambulance Inspection Checklist

### AMBULANCE OPERATION

#### Ambulance Equipment

Plugged in (electrical)............................ ___
Radio (operational).................................. ___
Telephone (operational).......................... ___
Emergency lights (operational)................ ___
Fuel (above ½ tank)................................ ___
Key (starts unit)...................................... ___
Tires (proper inflation, tread depth)........ ___
Inspection sticker (up to date)................ ___
Insurance card........................................ ___
IV warmer working (seasonal)................. ___
Windows clean......................................... ___
Unit clean (outside)................................. ___

#### Driver's Compartment

1–Hand light (6–12V)............................... ___
1–Spotlight (working)............................... ___
2–Protective gear (bunker coat, pants)...... ___
1–Emergency Response Guidebook......... ___
Driver's log book (mileage recorded)...... ___
Map/information book.............................. ___
Garage door opener................................ ___
Hospital map book................................... ___
Keys/gas card......................................... ___
Clean/trash removed............................... ___
Trip sheets box (with extra trip sheets)... ___
Completed patient paperwork/turned in.. ___
Accountability ring.................................... ___

### DRIVER-SIDE COMPARTMENTS

#### DA Compartment (Oxygen)

1–Oxygen cylinder M (500 psi)................. ___
1–Regulator (2,500–2,550 psi)................. ___
2–Padded board splints (54")................... ___
2–Padded board splints (36")................... ___
2–Padded board splints (15")................... ___
Reeves stretcher...................................... ___
Scoop stretcher........................................ ___
1–Fire extinguisher (2A:10BC, charged).... ___
1–Folding litter......................................... ___

#### DB Compartment (Tool)

Bag buster............................................... ___
2–Bunker helmets (hard hats).................. ___
2–Clear eye protection............................. ___
4–Disposable blankets (yellow)................ ___
**Access Equipment Toolbox ...... #** [___]

#### DC Compartment (Drawer)

2–Leather work gloves.............................. ___
3–Flares (30 min.).................................... ___
Tow strap................................................. ___
Battery jumper cables .............................. ___
Wheel simulator wrench........................... ___
2–Goggles................................................ ___

#### DD Compartment (VacuSplint)

1–SCBA/face mask (pressurized).............. ___
1–Vacu-splint mattress, with pump (child). ___
1–Vacu-splint mattress, with pump (child). ___
Vacu-splint kit (L, M, & S and pump)...... ___
Air-splint kit (6 pieces)............................ ___
1–Hand light (6–12V)............................... ___
**Primary Trauma Bag.................. #** [___]

### PASSENGER-SIDE COMPARTMENTS

#### PD Compartment (Backboard)

2–Long backboards (straps)..................... ___
1–KED (adult)........................................... ___
1–Pediatric immobilization board............. ___
1–Stair chair............................................ ___

#### PC Compartment (C-Collar)

2–CID blocks (with straps)........................ ___

#### Cervical Collar Bag

1–C-spine collar (infant)........................... ___
2–C-spine collars (pediatric).................... ___
2–C-spine collars (no-neck)..................... ___
2–C-spine collars (short).......................... ___
1–C-spine collar (regular)........................ ___
1–C-spine collar (tall).............................. ___
– OR –
3–C-spine collars (adjustable).................. ___

#### PB Compartment (Side Door)

2–Oxygen cylinder D (> 500 psi).............. ___
1–Oxygen cylinder D (on cot).................... ___
2–Flowmeter (1–25 lpm) with guard.......... ___
1–Wrench (as required)............................ ___
1–Folding litter/cot................................... ___
Unit clean/tidy (inside)............................. ___

#### PA Compartment (Drug Box)

1–Portable suction unit (& water)............. ___
1–Suction tubing...................................... ___
1–Rigid suction catheter.......................... ___
1–French suction catheter....................... ___
MAST with pump (adult).......................... ___
MAST with pump (child)........................... ___
**Pediatric Kit............................. #** [___]
**Auto Vent Kit............................. #** [___]
**Drug Box (locked).................... #** [___]

**Jonesville VFC Ambulance**  •  **111 Main Street**  •  **P.O. Box 978**  •  **Jonesville, MA 01803**  •  **(888) 555-1234**

**Figure 4-1** The EVO needs to document that the vehicle and all its systems are in proper operating condition. This is a sample page from a form used for this purpose.

Finally, as part of the exterior inspection, it is useful to check that all auxiliary equipment stored on the exterior of the vehicle is present and fully functional. Some outside compartment doors may not fully protect equipment from the elements, so steps must be taken to ensure cleanliness and regular maintenance of this equipment.

## Interior Compartments

The operator compartment (or cab) should be clean and neat. Electrical loads should be switched off, and all radios, audible warning devices (e.g., public address systems and sirens), and other necessary equipment should be present, functional, and accessible. For example, you should check that fire extinguishers are placed appropriately in both the driver and patient compartments and that their expiration date and gauge levels are appropriate, that the nozzles or hoses are intact and free of obstructions, that there is no rust or physical damage, and that the pins are intact and secure. It is essential for all equipment to be properly secured before the vehicle is in motion, as any unsecured equipment is likely to become a projectile and injure the patient or practitioners.

Next, check that the seatbelt and restraints operate correctly without binding. All belt webbing should be intact with no cuts, and buckles should easily release when activated and close securely. Many emergency vehicles are equipped with air ride seats, which are adjustable for height, position, and angle. These seats should be adjusted for optimal comfort and vehicle control.

All mirrors should be properly adjusted for the maximum field of vision so that the vehicle operator can see down the length of the vehicle. Convex mirrors should be adjusted so the insides of the mirrors have the edge of the emergency vehicle as a reference. If the mirrors have a heat control, the operator should be familiar with this function. Examine the lights in the interior to ensure they are functional, and check for signs of internal moisture.

The EVO should also examine all gauges and meters to ensure they are fully functional and within an acceptable range for safe vehicle operation. The gauges and meters that should be checked are described as follows:

- The *fuel gauge* shows the amount of fuel in the tank. The vehicle should have an adequate level of fuel to respond to a call. If the vehicle has dual tanks, note which tank the gauge is reading and switch to the other tank to check the level in it as well. Experience with a particular vehicle will provide the operator with functional knowledge of its fuel range.
- The *oil pressure gauge* indicates the delivery pressure of lubricating oil to the engine.
- The *air pressure gauge* shows the amount of air in the air brake system. Typically, these systems have multiple tanks with safety valves installed to prevent catastrophic loss of air. Many systems will have two different-colored indicator needles for front and rear pressure systems installed in a single gauge or multiple gauges.
- The *coolant temperature gauge* indicates the temperature of the engine coolant.
- The *speedometer* indicates the speed of the vehicle when moving.
- The *odometer* records miles traveled.
- The *hour meter* registers the number of hours the engine has been running.
- The *tachometer* registers the speed of the engine in rpm.
- The *voltmeter* (or ammeter) indicates battery voltage and shows if the alternator is charging the system.

Some of these, like the speedometer, cannot be easily checked during daily inspections; frequency of testing should be outlined in your maintenance SOPs. Any warnings that are indicated should be reported as required by your company policy.

## Mechanical Components and Systems

Your ambulance is a machine that is designed to perform specific functions. As with any other machine, it can be more efficiently operated and maintained if you understand its various mechanical components and systems. Ambulances have many of the same mechanical components as your personal vehicle, plus some extras.

# Engine

The power for operating the vehicle is provided by the **engine**, which in most cases runs on either gasoline or diesel. The engine creates power by combusting fuel in cylinders that are within the block (inner core) of the engine. This combustion process pushes pistons in each cylinder that are attached to a rotating crankshaft. The pressure of the combustion on the top of the piston pushes it down and the combination of all of the pistons moving in synchronization causes the crankshaft to rotate. Most ambulances have a tachometer gauge that tells the operator how many revolutions per minute (rpm) the crankshaft is turning—usually between about 500 and 3,000, depending on the vehicle.

The engine must have lubrication between the pistons and the cylinder walls to allow the pistons to move smoothly inside the cylinder. The engine oil, which is held in a pan at the bottom of the engine and is pumped through the engine as it is running, provides this lubrication. If the amount of engine oil gets too low, friction will build up between the pistons and the cylinder walls and may cause a piston to lock up inside the cylinder, ruining the engine.

The exhaust gases from the internal combustion are removed from each cylinder by the revolution of the crankshaft pushing the piston back up and the gases above the piston out through the open exhaust valve. These gases are routed through pipes located on the sides of the engine to the exhaust system underneath the vehicle. The exhaust system also includes catalytic converters that reduce the pollutants in the exhaust gases and mufflers that reduce the noise caused by the escaping gases.

The exhaust system gets very hot during operation and remains hot for quite a while after the engine is turned off. The engine exhaust gases contain carbon monoxide, which is odorless, but very deadly, when inhaled, so the vehicle should never be left running inside an enclosed area without adequate ventilation.

The internal combustion of the engine produces a significant amount of heat, which can also damage the engine. To avoid overheating, the engine has a cooling system that uses engine coolant to circulate around the outsides of the cylinders (within the engine block) absorbing the heat of the engine. This coolant is pumped through the engine and then through hoses to the radiator located in front of the engine. As the coolant flows through tubes inside the radiator, the air passing across the radiator around these tubes removes the heat it has absorbed from the engine. Once the heat has been removed, the coolant is again circulated through the engine to repeat the process. The coolant, which in most cases is a combination of water and other chemicals such as ethylene glycol, is very efficient at removing heat without freezing inside the engine if the outside temperature gets too cold and the engine is not running. The coolant often reaches temperatures in excess of 200°F during operation and creates pressures of around 15 to 20 pounds per square inch (psi) inside the cooling system. Most ambulances will have a gauge that indicates the temperature of the coolant. If the coolant temperature gets too high, the vehicle should be stopped and the engine turned off to prevent permanent engine damage due to overheating.

On the front of the engine, there are often several devices mounted that have pulleys on them. One or more rubber belts to the crankshaft of the engine attach these pulleys. This arrangement allows the rotation of the engine to drive these devices, such as an alternator for producing electricity for the vehicle, a power steering pump that provides hydraulic assistance for the steering of the vehicle, and an air-conditioning compressor that allows cool air to circulate through the unit in hot weather. In addition, on some units there may be an air compressor that provides compressed air if the vehicle is equipped with an air brake system. As you can imagine, if these belts break, the devices they operate will stop functioning, putting the unit out of service.

The engine compartment should be clean (**Figure 4-2**). A clean compartment allows for the detection of new leaks or problems and helps the engine stay cool. Any belts should be intact and snug, with no cracks, cuts, or damage. Hoses should be properly attached and show no signs of leakage. Always maintain clearance from belts and fans while performing daily inspections. Items such as jewelry, long hair, and loose clothing can be caught between moving parts. Also, most vehicles have radiator fans that are powered by the vehicle's battery and can turn on and off unexpectedly (even with the engine off).

In the engine compartment, you should check the levels of oil and coolant. To check the oil level, first ensure that the engine has been turned off for at least 5 minutes and the vehicle is on level ground so that the oil reading will be accurate (oil distributes throughout the engine when it is running and then drains back into the oil pan, and parking on an incline could cause the oil to shift, altering the measurable level). Next, locate the dipstick and remove it, wipe it off, and reinsert it. Completely reseat the dipstick and then remove it again and read the oil level in relation to the markings on the stick (**Figure 4-3**). The engine dipstick typically has marks indicating whether the oil level is sufficient or additional oil needs to be added. Depending on the engine, anywhere from 1 quart to 1 gallon may be required to bring the level from low to full. When adding oil, ensure that it is the proper type and viscosity required for the engine of your specific vehicle per the owner's manual. This

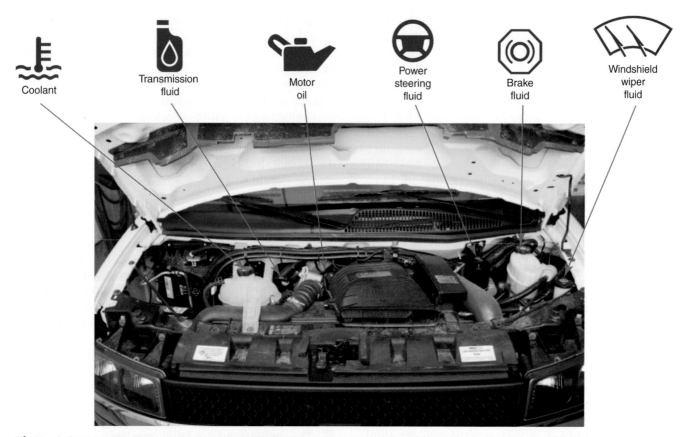

**Figure 4-2** The symbols for coolant, transmission fluid, motor oil, power steering fluid, brake fluid, and windshield wiper fluid, and their respective locations in a typical ambulance engine compartment.

Photo: © Jones & Bartlett Learning. Photographed by Darren Stahlman. Coolant Icon: © Gercen/Shutterstock. Motor Oil Icon: © Liudmyla Marykon/Shutterstock. Brake Fluid Icon: © A Aleksii/Shutterstock. Transmission, Power Steering, Windshield Wiper Fluid Icon: © Alexandr III/Shutterstock.

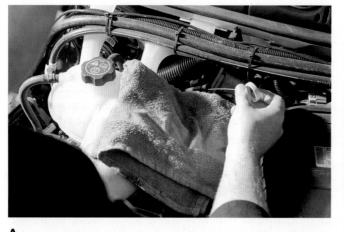

**A**

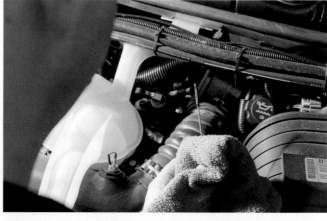

**B**

**Figure 4-3** When performing an oil check, you must first wipe off and fully reseat the dipstick. You then **(A)** remove it a second time and **(B)** check the oil level.

© Jones & Bartlett Learning. Photographed by Darren Stahlman.

information is also found on the oil fill cap of most new engines. If oil is leaking, you may notice pools of fluid under the engine in the color of the oil, which is typically golden or black. Conduct these checks and refill oil only if it is within your company's policy.

To check the coolant, ensure that the engine has been turned off for at least 5 minutes for safety. Removing the radiator cap when the engine is hot is rarely recommended, as it can easily release coolant as steam and cause a boil over of the coolant and possible injury. Most newer vehicles have see-through coolant reservoirs with hot and cold markings, making it easy to visualize coolant levels and unnecessary to remove the radiator cap.

## Electrical System

The **electrical system** provides all electrical energy for vehicle operation and takes on heavy demands in the modern emergency vehicle. Although efforts have been made through the federal specifications to limit the electrical demands of emergency vehicles, they are still heavy. There are several key components of the electrical system:

- **Alternators** produce current for the electrical system and are powered by an engine-driven belt.
- **Batteries** store electrical energy to help start the vehicle and provide a backup power source should the alternator fail; they typically provide only a few minutes of power under these circumstances.
- **Inverters** convert direct current (DC) power from the vehicle's electrical system to alternating current (AC) power—the same as household current—to enable the operation of hospital-type equipment, such as suction units and cardiac monitors, during transport or the ability to use an AC-powered accessory charger for charging cell phones in the ambulance.

Because of the high electrical demand in emergency vehicles, they can occasionally suffer from electrical problems. Jumper cables may be useful to "jump-start" a vehicle when the battery has died. Care should be taken to clearly understand the procedure for jump-starting a vehicle, and eye protection should be worn when performing this task. Since jump-starting a vehicle can result in electrical spikes to the system, all electronic devices on the emergency vehicle should be turned off when performing the procedure. Always follow your service's SOPs, since some agencies do not allow crew members to perform any mechanical procedures on the vehicles.

## Drivetrain

The drivetrain is the entire system of components that provide power to the wheels, including the transmission, transfer case, driveshafts, and differential.

The engine is connected to a **transmission** that is located behind the engine and that uses internal gears to convert the revolutions of the engine to slower revolutions that are required by the vehicle wheels as it is accelerating. As the speed of the vehicle increases or decreases, the transmission allows the revolutions of the wheels to change within the normal range of rpm of the engine by applying different gears. At slow speeds, a lower gear is used, and higher gears are applied as the vehicle reaches higher speeds. The transmission must have constant lubrication for the gears as well as for the internal hydraulics, which shift the gears when appropriate. Transmission fluid is a special type of hydraulic fluid. It is usually dark red in color and rarely causes problems unless a seal at one end of the transmission fails, allowing the fluid to leak out.

Most ambulances have automatic transmissions. New technology has allowed for the design of automatic transmissions to handle the heavier weight of emergency vehicles. These transmissions are hydraulic systems, which require adequate levels of fluid to function properly. Additionally, they are usually electronic, requiring a properly functioning electrical system to select the proper shift patterns.

Newer transmissions are being designed to utilize computer programming to prevent damage to the unit. For example, if the vehicle is rolling forward, the computer would ensure that the transmission would not shift into reverse before the vehicle was brought to a complete stop. Designs have also been developed to ensure that the vehicle cannot be placed into drive unless the vehicle is idling.

The transmission revolutions are transmitted to the wheels through a driveshaft and a rear-end gear that changes the direction of rotation and causes the wheels to turn. There are rarely any problems with this part of the drivetrain, but fluid leaking from the rear-end gear would be cause for concern. The rear-end gear, also known as the rear differential, is in the middle of the rear axle (the shaft going from side to side between the rear wheels). If you find fluid (usually dark gray to black) leaking from this area, the unit should be put out of service for repair.

Routine preventive maintenance for the drivetrain includes checking transmission and power steering fluid levels. The transmission is a hydraulic system, and the dipstick is commonly marked with hot and cold notations. Some vehicles require checks with the transmission in neutral, and some in park, but almost always with the engine running. Make sure the parking brake is applied if the engine is in neutral. The procedure for checking the power steering fluid is the same as for the engine oil (just using a different dipstick and with the engine running). The power steering is also a hydraulic system. It is commonly checked with a dipstick installed on the cap and marked with hot and cold notations. The power steering fluid level should be checked with the engine off. Many power steering units simply use automatic transmission fluid, but make sure to follow the manufacturer's recommendations, found in the owner's manual and company policy.

## Braking System

Historically, the **braking system** has been one of the most abused systems on an ambulance. Since most ambulances have a greater gross vehicle weight rating than a typical passenger car, these heavier vehicles are outfitted to handle additional stress and strain. Some vehicles are also equipped with auxiliary braking devices, which slow the vehicle by acting on the driveshaft, transmission, or engine. These devices normally act on the rear wheels and can be set to varying degrees of deceleration. However, caution should be used when using these devices on slick roads where they may cause the rear of the vehicle to skid.

There are several different types of brakes used in emergency vehicles. **Drum brakes** have a circular wheel hub with two semicircular brake shoes as shown in **Figure 4-4**. When the brake pedal is pressed, a piston spreads the brake shoes outward against the drum, using friction to slow the vehicle. Release of the brake pedal allows springs to return the brake shoes to their resting position. **Disc brakes** are designed with a disc and a brake caliper, with brake pads on the inside of the caliper (**Figure 4-5**). The caliper is installed over the disc. Pressing on the brake pedal causes the caliper to compress the brake pads against the rotating disc, slowing the vehicle.

**Hydraulic brakes** use fluid to charge and activate the brakes. When you step on the brake pedal, fluid is compressed through the system and the pressure is applied to the brake pads or shoes, forcing them out against the rotor or drum. If fluid is lost due to a leak or other means, the system cannot pressurize and the result is complete brake failure.

**Air brakes** have the same task as hydraulic systems but function differently and require different maintenance. In a triple-valve air brake system, the air holds the brake pads away from the wheel, allowing it to turn freely. Depressing the brake pedal releases air from a chamber to activate the brake system instead of fluid pushing against the system. The parking system on air brakes also works differently from a hydraulic system. The park position on air brakes allows a mechanical spring to activate the brakes and holds the vehicle in place. This design enables a vehicle with common noncritical slow leaks in the air system to be parked for an indefinite amount of time. A certain amount of air pressure, typically about 60 psi, is required to deactivate the spring system on the brakes. Their deactivation allows the parking brake to be released so the vehicle can roll. It is important to note that at any time while operating this type of vehicle, if the air pressure becomes lower than the spring pressure, the springs will take over, locking the brakes and causing the vehicle to skid to a stop.

**Antilock brakes** are a type of brake system that uses a computer system to detect wheel lockup and briefly reduce braking action to that particular wheel, allowing rotation and directional control to be maintained. Antilock brakes do not necessarily decrease stopping distance, but they protect the wheels from locking up and prevent the turning of the vehicle. Antilock brakes are especially useful on slippery surfaces. Caution should be exercised

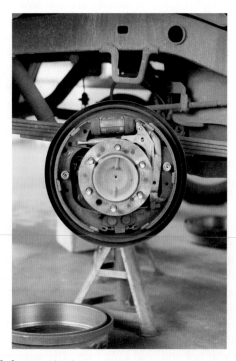

**Figure 4-4** Drum brakes.
© Toa55/iStock/Getty Images

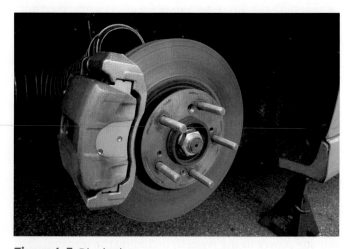

**Figure 4-5** Disc brakes.
© schlol/iStock/Getty Images

when using an antilock braking system on uneven roads, such as cobblestone or gravel, since braking distance can be increased.

Since inspection of the mechanical brake components requires the removal of the wheels, this process is not included in daily routine vehicle inspection. Brake systems should, however, be checked by qualified mechanics on a regular schedule. If the vehicle has hydraulic brakes, the brake fluid should be checked routinely. Most new vehicles are equipped with a see-through reservoir where the level of this fluid can be visualized. If the brake fluid level appears low, notify a supervisor. Low brake fluid usually indicates worn brakes, which will require the unit to be out of service for maintenance. Low brake fluid may also be caused by leaks, so make sure to check underneath the reservoir as well as behind each wheel for puddles of brake fluid. If you discover brake fluid leaks, this should also be reason to put the unit out of service. Never simply add fluid and continue driving the vehicle; doing so could lead to catastrophic brake failure. Some newer brake fluids are hydroscopic (absorb moisture), so opening the reservoir daily simply introduces unwanted moisture into the system. This problem can be avoided by simply looking through the reservoir to gauge the level of the brake fluid.

Air brakes should be tested daily by performing the "ALSAPS method":

- *Air brake leakage test.* Depress the brake pedal and hold it. There should be an immediate reduction of air, but not more than 10 psi. Continue to depress the pedal for 1 minute. The system should not lose more than 2 psi in that time.
- *Low air warning test.* Turn on the power supply, but do not start the vehicle. Begin fanning (rapidly pressing and releasing) the brakes until pressure drops and the warning light and buzzer activate. Note that pressure on the gauge should be around 70 psi.
- *Spring brake test.* With the vehicle on level ground, push the parking brake in. Begin fanning the brake pedal until the parking brake "pops" out. Note that pressure on the gauge should be around 40 psi.
- *Air compressor cutoff test.* Start the engine and monitor the air compressor gauge. The air compressor should cut off around 125 psi. This process should be completed in under 2 minutes.
- *Parking brake test.* With the vehicle still running and the parking brake on, shift into gear and gently step on the accelerator, checking that the parking brake is holding.
- *Service brake test.* With the vehicle in drive and your foot on the brake, release the parking brake and allow the vehicle to roll slowly 15 to 50 feet. Depress the brake and stop the vehicle. The service brake is functional.

If the brakes are used heavily during a trip, you may notice a burning smell coming from the area of the wheels. This odor is caused by the brake pad material overheating and is a sign that the brakes have been pushed to their limit. Occasionally under extremely heavy use, brakes can fail, resulting in an inability to stop the vehicle. This true emergency can often be avoided by limiting heavy use of the brakes through reasonable and careful driving.

## Tires

Tires on the ambulance are expected to be durable and perform well at high speeds. They should be inspected at the beginning of each shift, examining for proper inflation, adequate tread, and any signs of damage such as cuts, cracks, or uneven wear. You will need to check the tire inflation pressure to ensure that it falls within the manufacturer's recommendations for the specific vehicle type. These recommendations are normally located on a sticker inside the driver's door, the door jamb, or the glove box door (**Figure 4-6**). Because the manufacturer recommendations for tire pressures are based on the gross vehicle weight rating, they may vary from the maximum pressure listed on the tire. It is important to follow the vehicle manufacturer's guidelines, while not exceeding the tire manufacturer's stated limits.

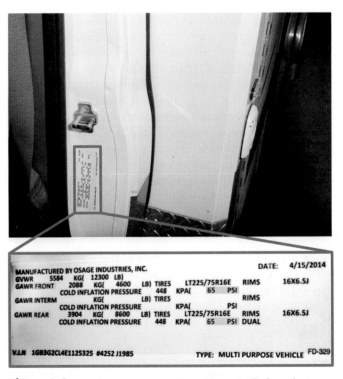

**Figure 4-6** The tire pressure tag (inset) is typically found on the inside of the driver's door.

© Jones & Bartlett Learning. Photographed by Darren Stahlman.

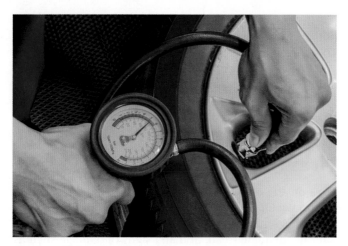

**Figure 4-7** Check tire pressure regularly.
© Shine Nucha/Shutterstock

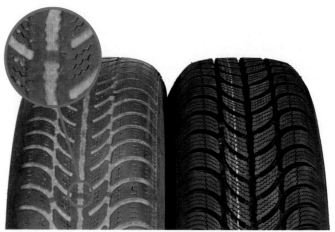

**Figure 4-8** Prominent wear bars (inset) indicate that the tread is worn and that the tire must be replaced.
© algre/iStock/Getty Images

To check the tire pressure, you will need a high-quality tire pressure gauge. Tire pressure gauges come with different measurement ranges. Typical car gauges measure pressure up to only 50 psi, but commercial vehicle gauges may have a range of greater than 100 psi. Make sure your gauge is appropriate for the task at hand. It is important to note that tire pressure increases when the tires are hot, so it is best to check tire pressure after the vehicle has been idle for at least 3 hours. To check the tire pressure, first remove the protective cap from the air valve, then firmly press the gauge inlet against the **valve stem** to prevent air loss (**Figure 4-7**). Read the measurement on the gauge and adjust air pressure as needed by adding air with an air compressor hose and nozzle or releasing excess air by compressing the needle inside the valve stem. Do *not* let air out of a tire that has just been driven or is hot; doing so can cause the tire to be underinflated when it cools. Note that reducing the air pressure is not usually necessary unless someone has previously overinflated the tire. Make sure all tires are inflated equally. Unequal inflation will lead to poor vehicle handling as well as a higher likelihood of tire failure. Remember that changes in weather and barometric pressure can change the pressure of a tire.

> **SAFETY TIP**
>
> Proper tire inflation is important to the safe handling of the emergency vehicle. Automatic tire pressure gauges will be included in those ambulances built or updated to meet NFPA 1917, *Standard for Automotive Ambulances.*

Wear bars are small portions of rubber that lie underneath the tire's surface and are perpendicular to the tread (**Figure 4-8**). As the tread slowly wears away, the wear bars become more prominent until they become level with the tire's tread. When this occurs, it is mandatory to change the tire since the sipes are not deep enough to channel away water. Actual tread depth measurements are tire specific, but commercial tire requirements of 4/32 in for steering tires and 2/32 in for rear tires can be used as a guideline. (For further information on treads, see the section on hydroplaning in Chapter 4.)

## Suspension System

The **suspension system** is what supports the vehicle above the drivetrain. Most ambulances are equipped with heavy-duty suspension systems to withstand the rigors of emergency use. Suspension systems have improved greatly in recent years, and many newer vehicles have air suspension systems that provide a smooth and comfortable ride. The suspension system in newer vehicles may also lower the rear of the vehicle to make it easier to get in and out of the patient compartment. Combined with stabilization systems, which reduce vehicle body roll (a tendency for the top of the vehicle to lean outward) in curves, improved suspension systems have made the vehicles much more comfortable and safer to use. Since the suspension system is located under the vehicle, it should be inspected by qualified mechanics on a regular schedule.

## Heating and Air-Conditioning System

In accordance with federal guidelines, all ambulances used to transport patients must have adequate heating and cooling systems to maintain a temperature of

68–78°F in the patient compartment. Most emergency vehicle heating systems work off the vehicle coolant system. A series of hoses channel hot coolant to the patient module where a fan and radiator arrangement introduces heated air into the patient compartment. Electronic or mechanical valves controlled by a thermostat system regulate the temperature. Some vehicles are also equipped with electrical or mechanical valves under the hood that may cut off the flow of coolant to the patient module when it is not needed due to warm external temperatures. Most ambulance air-conditioning systems have one compressor and condenser to cool the cab and a secondary compressor and condenser system to cool the patient compartment.

### SAFETY TIP

While not required, it is a good idea to maintain a temperature of 68–78°F in the patient compartment, so the area is at the proper temperature when the need to transport a patient arises.

## Exhaust System

The **exhaust system** of the vehicle should be intact and functional, channeling all exhaust gases safely out the side or the rear of the vehicle. It is important to note where the exhaust exits the vehicle and to avoid aligning the exhaust output with the area of injured patients at a scene. Remember that the carbon monoxide in exhaust gases is colorless and odorless and can cause serious problems if it leaks into the ambulance. To avoid this situation, some ambulances are equipped with carbon

### OPERATOR INCIDENT

During the morning checkout, Danny was behind schedule and completed the inspection sheet in a hurry. Later that day, another EMT, Carl, was responding to a call and was unable to contact anyone on the radio. He had to resort to the unit's cell phone to get in touch with the hospital. After wheeling the patient into the hospital on the stretcher, he returned to the vehicle, but the engine would not start. He tried to turn the unit's headlights on to determine if there was a problem with the battery and discovered that the headlights weren't working either. He opened the hood of the unit and noticed the alternator belt lying beneath the radiator. The alternator belt could have been easily replaced if only Danny had done a thorough vehicle inspection.

monoxide detectors in the patient module. A qualified mechanic should regularly inspect the exhaust system, which is located underneath the unit.

## Preventive Maintenance

Most EMS services require a daily inspection of the vehicle. This inspection is important to maintain the vehicle, helping it to last longer and perform more efficiently, and also to reduce potential liability from a failed vehicle due to a defective or damaged component. **Preventive maintenance**, regularly inspecting and servicing the vehicle, helps reduce equipment downtime and repair costs. It is more economical to schedule servicing and replacement at regular intervals than to pay for unexpected repairs. Preventive maintenance may be performed at intervals determined by the vehicle's mileage or a certain amount of time. For example, engine oil changes are not dependent on the vehicle's mileage as in personal vehicles, since emergency vehicles typically spend more time in idle (i.e., the engine is running, but this engine work is not registered by the odometer); however, tire inspection and maintenance should be based on the vehicle's mileage rather than a designated amount of time.

Maintenance schedules may vary based on the severity of the problem. Any problems that affect the safety of the vehicle (e.g., a cut in a tire or brake issues) should be addressed immediately. Less critical problems (e.g., a nonoperative clearance light) may be repaired during scheduled routine maintenance.

## Road Performance

Some EMS systems include road performance as part of vehicle inspections; this should be performed by a qualified mechanic as part of their required routine inspections since certain problems can be detected only by driving the vehicle. If your service requires this test by a mechanic, you should take note if any the following occur during regular use and report to your supervisor:

- The steering wheel should be properly aligned and should turn smoothly, accurately directing the vehicle with little play.
- There should be no unexpected noises. For example, a high-pitched squealing noise may indicate a worn or loose power steering belt.
- The brake pedal should be firm, and the vehicle should slow in proportion to pedal pressure.
- The brakes should stop the vehicle evenly without pulling to the left or right and should perform consistently, even during repeated stops.
- The vehicle should accelerate with smooth engine operation and no skipping.

# Relevant Guidelines and Organizations

Several standards and organizations provide useful guidelines and resources for emergency vehicle inspection and maintenance. Vehicle operators should be familiar with NFPA 1071, *Standard for Emergency Vehicle Technician Professional Qualifications*. This standard outlines the minimum job performance requirements for a person qualified as an emergency vehicle technician who is engaged in the inspection, diagnosis, maintenance, repair, and testing of an emergency vehicle. While this standard is intended for the fire service, it does have some useful information that can be applied to all providers of emergency services. In addition, NFPA 1911, *Standard for the Inspection, Maintenance, Testing, and Retirement of In-Service Automotive Fire Apparatus*, provides minimum requirements for a preventive maintenance program for fire apparatus and sets a standard for many emergency personnel and agency SOPs.

NFPA 1917, *Standard for Automotive Ambulances*, is becoming the new standard for ambulance design and construction and is steadily replacing the KKK-A-1822F specifications for ambulances built on or after January 1, 2013.

The Emergency Vehicle Technician (EVT) Certification Commission, Inc., is a nonprofit corporation that seeks to improve the quality of emergency vehicle service and repair. This organization offers a certification program for vehicle technicians recognizing the training and experience they have in the service and repair of emergency vehicles. Automotive Service Excellence (ASE) is another nonprofit certification agency that tests professionals' vehicle repair and service abilities.

When your inspection or use of your emergency vehicle reveals a problem, you should report the problem in accordance with your chain of command and the SOPs within your agency. You should not drive a vehicle that you feel is unsafe. Remember that as the EVO, you will be held responsible for any collisions or injuries that occur. It is the employer's responsibility, in accordance with the Occupational Safety and Health Act (OSH), to provide a safe work environment, free from recognized hazards that can cause death or serious harm. States may have additional standards and different enforcement policies. NFPA 1911 allows the authority having jurisdiction to define defects considered unsafe for vehicle operation and outlines the responsibility to remove the vehicle from service.

## SUMMARY

- As the EVO, you are generally charged with making sure your unit is mechanically ready prior to your initial operation of the vehicle.
- You should be familiar with the mechanical operation of your vehicle and potential problems that might routinely occur.
- You should be very familiar with the daily inspection checklist for your vehicle and complete it in a thorough and responsible manner on every shift.
- You should be able to determine which maintenance you can reliably perform, and which maintenance needs to be referred to a qualified mechanic, based on your company's policies.
- The EVO should mark out of service any unit believed to be unsafe, pending repair.

## GLOSSARY

**air brakes** A braking system that uses air as a medium for applying the brakes.

**alternators** Electromechanical devices that convert mechanical energy to electrical energy in the form of alternating current; automotive alternators use a set of rectifiers mechanical energy to electrical energy in the form of alternating current; automotive alternators use a set of rectifiers to convert alternating current to direct current to charge the vehicle batteries.

**antilock brakes** A computerized braking system that prevents wheel lockup, helping the vehicle maintain directional control.

**batteries** Devices that chemically store electrical energy; they are generally used for starting the vehicle and short-term electrical use.

**braking system** The entire system that allows the vehicle operator to stop the vehicle by applying pressure to the vehicle's brake pedal.

**disc brakes** A braking system designed with a disc and a brake caliper installed over the disc.

**drum brakes** A braking system that has a circular wheel hub with two semicircular brake shoes installed inside.

**electrical system** The system that generates and maintains electrical energy required for vehicle operation as well as for patient care activities.

**engine** A device that provides the mechanical motive force for propelling a vehicle and powering its subsystems.

**exhaust system** The system for removing dangerous exhaust gases from the engine.

**hydraulic brakes** A braking system that uses fluid to charge and activate the brakes.

**inverters** Electrical devices that convert direct current to alternating current; they provide 110-volt current.

**preventive maintenance** Scheduled servicing, inspection, or replacement of specific items in the vehicle to reduce potential problems.

**suspension system** The system that supports the vehicle and allows it to absorb the impact from bumpy roads without affecting the ride inside the cab and patient compartment.

**transmission** A device that provides speed and torque conversions from the engine to the wheels using gear ratios; it reduces the higher engine speed to the slower wheel speed, increasing torque in the process.

**valve stem** An opening to the valve that admits air to a tire and automatically closes to seal in pressure

## ADDITIONAL RESOURCES

Automotive Service Excellence, http://www.ase.com

Emergency Vehicle Technician Certification Commission, http://www.evtcc.org

NFPA 1071, *Standard for Emergency Vehicle Technician Professional Qualification*

NFPA 1911, *Standard for the Inspection, Maintenance, Testing, and Retirement of In-Service Automotive Fire Apparatus*

NFPA 1917, *Standard for Automotive Ambulances*

## REFERENCES

U.S. Fire Administration, Federal Emergency Management Agency. (2014). *Emergency vehicle safety initiative*. FEMA FA-336. Retrieved from https://www.usfa.fema.gov/downloads/pdf/publications/fa_336.pdf

# CHAPTER 5

# Maneuvering Your Vehicle

## OBJECTIVES

**5.1** Identify gross vehicle weight ratings for the five types of ambulances.

**5.2** Explain how size and weight affect vehicle operation and control.

**5.3** Describe how physical factors such as friction, gravity, inertia, and energy affect vehicle operation and performance.

**5.4** Discuss concerns related to visibility and quality of ride.

**5.5** Explain how road construction and shape affect vehicle control.

**5.6** Calculate following distance and know how to maintain a safety cushion around the ambulance.

**5.7** Explain the potential hazards and cautions for driving in inclement weather.

**5.8** Discuss safety considerations for specific vehicle maneuvers such as braking and stopping, negotiating curves and turns, changing lanes, backing, parking, and crossing intersections.

**5.9** Explain why many intersections are being redesigned as roundabouts.

## SCENARIO

When John left his supervisor's office, he was mad. His partner had complained that John's rough driving made it difficult for him to provide effective patient care in the ambulance, while John thought his ability to operate an emergency vehicle was just fine. After John cooled down, he recalled previous comments from his coworkers about his driving. He had written them off, assuming they were just the kind of normal banter that exists around the station. Now he realized that maybe people had been trying to subtly give him a message.

John went back to his supervisor and discussed the situation again. Although John had kept up with his continuing education and always attended in-service emergency vehicle operator (EVO) training sessions, together John and his supervisor decided that perhaps he needed a bit more specialized training to deal with this issue. John's supervisor made arrangements for him and his partner to use a nearby parking lot for a training session where they changed roles. John pretended to attend to a patient in the rear of the ambulance,

*(continues)*

# Types of Ambulances

The U.S. General Services Administration identifies minimum requirements for new ambulances that are fully built from the chassis up. These requirements are outlined in a document known as KKK-A-1822F, which describes ambulances that are authorized to display the Star of Life symbol as seen in **Figure 5-1**. The document establishes minimum specifications, performance parameters, and essential criteria for ambulance design to provide standardization and ensure that ambulances are properly constructed. Note that the KKK-A-1822F specifications are designed as a checklist for the governmental body buying the ambulance, not as a method to ensure crew or patient safety; compliance with this document is voluntary and the manufacturer does not have to maintain a standard. However, in recent years, due in part to the adoption of NFPA 1917, *Standard for Automotive Ambulances*, manufacturers have voluntarily taken on a more proactive stance in developing safer, stronger, and more ergonomically designed vehicles.

There are five different types of ambulances, based on gross vehicle weight and design (**Table 5-1**). All vehicles have a **gross vehicle weight rating (GVWR)**, which represents the manufacturer's maximum allowable weight limit of the vehicle. On Star of Life ambulances,

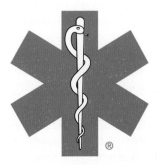

**Figure 5-1** The Star of Life symbol demonstrates that a vehicle meets federal standards for quality performance.

Courtesy of the U.S. Department of Transportation, National Highway Traffic Safety Administration.

| Table 5-1 Gross Vehicle Weight Ratings | |
|---|---|
| **Ambulance Type** | **Gross Vehicle Weight Rating (pounds)** |
| Type 1 | 10,001 to 14,000 |
| Type 1 additional duty (AD) | > 14,001 |
| Type 2 | 9,201 to 10,000 |
| Type 3 | 10,001 to 14,000 |
| Type 3 AD | > 14,001 |

© Jones & Bartlett Learning

| CERTIFIED "STAR OF LIFE" AMBULANCE | | |
|---|---|---|
| MFG BY _____ | DATE OF MANUFACTURE MO, YR_____ | |
| ADDRESS _____ | | |
| CITY _____ STATE___ ZIP _____ | | |
| This Ambulance conforms to Federal Specification KKK-A-1822 in effect on the date of manufacture shown above. | | |
| AMBULANCE IDENTIFICATION NUMBER _____ TYPE - CLASS - FLOOR PLAN - SERIAL NO. | | |
| CURB WEIGHT | PAYLOAD MAX | GROSS WT. MAX |
| _____ kg/lbs. | _____ kg/lbs. | _____ kg/lbs. |

**Figure 5-2** A sample label, featuring the GVWR, for a certified Star of Life ambulance.

Reproduced from the Federal Specification for the "Star-of-Life Ambulance," KKK-A-1822E modular box for patient care.

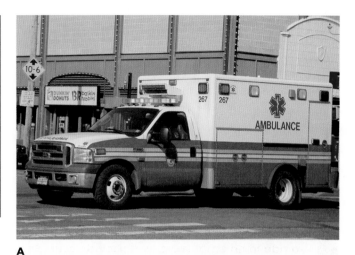

**A**

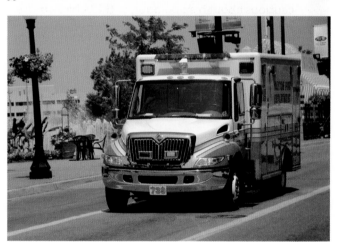

**B**

**Figure 5-3** **A.** Type 1 ambulance. **B.** Type 1 AD ambulance.
**A:** © Leonard Zhukovsky/Shutterstock; **B:** © imac/Alamy Stock Photo

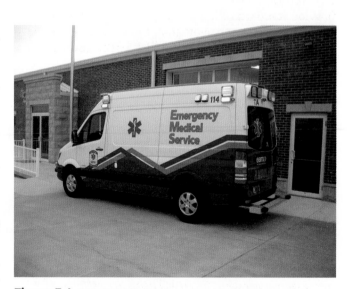

**Figure 5-4** Type 2 ambulance.
© Osage Ambulances

this rating is documented on a specification tag (**Figure 5-2**). It is illustrated by the letters GVWR and may be divided into front and rear axle weights, with a total vehicle weight illustrated. This total exemplifies the fact that neither the front nor the rear axle should be overloaded, and the complete vehicle needs to fall within the GVWR. If it is exceeded, the manufacturer will not back the vehicle's warranty and the vehicle will not perform safely.

Type 1 ambulances have a GVWR of 10,001 to 14,000 pounds (**Figure 5-3A**). The design is a cab chassis furnished with a replaceable modular ambulance body, in which patient care is performed. A small pass-through (a minimum size of 150 square inches) is required between the front of the patient module and the rear of the driver compartment. Type 1 additional duty (AD) ambulances have an increased GVWR of 14,001 pounds or more (**Figure 5-3B**).

Type 2 ambulances have a GVWR of 9,201 to 10,000 pounds. They are standard long-wheelbase vans that are customized to meet emergency vehicle and patient care specifications (**Figure 5-4**). They are typically designed with a raised roof to meet patient compartment requirements.

Type 3 ambulances have a GVWR of 10,001 to 14,000 pounds (**Figure 5-5A**). The design is a cutaway van with an integrated modular body. This vehicle style has a required walk-through opening between the driver compartment and the patient module. If a door is included, it must have the 150-square-inch window at the driver's eye level. Type 3 AD ambulances have an increased GVWR of 14,001 pounds or more (**Figure 5-5B**).

The term **payload** refers to the amount of weight the vehicle can carry within its GVWR ratings. The GVWR is the total permissible weight, which includes the weight of the vehicle, equipment, fuel, and personnel. For example, if the GVWR of the ambulance is 14,000 pounds and the empty vehicle weighs 11,000 pounds, no more than 3,000 pounds of equipment and personnel can be carried at any given time.

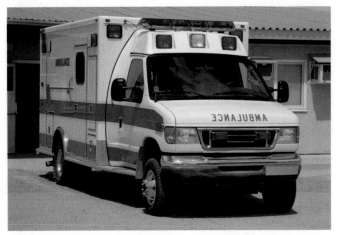

**A**

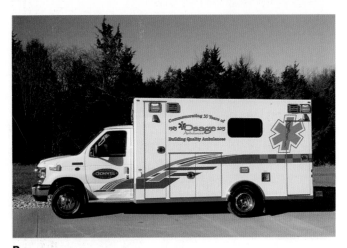

**B**

**Figure 5-5** **A.** Type 3 ambulance. **B.** Type 3 AD ambulance.

**A:** © HHakim/iStock/Getty Images; **B:** Courtesy of Cromwell Emergency Vehicles, Inc.

## Ambulance Crash Testing

The National Institute for Occupational Safety and Health (NIOSH) and the Department of Homeland Security's Science and Technology Directorate partnered with other federal agencies and the ambulance manufacturing industry to conduct ambulance crash testing to reduce and eliminate crash-related injuries and deaths to EMS practitioners in the patient compartment. These dynamic crash tests contributed to the development of 10 test methods published by the Society of Automotive Engineers (SAE). The test methods fall into the categories outlined in **Table 5-2**.

To watch a series of videos to learn more about the many changes impacting ambulance design, testing, and manufacturing, go to www.cdc.gov/niosh/topics/ems/videos.html.

## Physical Factors Affecting Vehicle Operation and Performance

Several physical factors affect a vehicle's operation and performance. **Friction** is the resistance of one object to sliding over another. Soft, tacky materials have a higher degree of friction than hard, smooth materials. For example, rubber has more friction on asphalt than it does on wet ice. **Gravity** is the force that pulls objects toward the earth, resulting in what we know as weight. Weight gives the vehicle the ability to produce friction against a road surface.

| Table 5-2 Ambulance Crash Test Methods | | |
|---|---|---|
| **Methods: Exterior** | **Title** | **Consists of** |
| | SAE J2917 | Crash pulse from frontal impact |
| | SAE J3057 | Modular body (or box style) roof crush test |
| | SAE J3044 | Crash pulse from rear impact |
| | SAE J2956 | Crash pulse from side impact |
| **Methods: Interior** | SAE J3026 | EMS practitioner seating and restraints |
| | SAE J3027 | Patient cot, floor mount, and restraint system integrity test |
| | SAE J3043 | Ambulance equipment mount devices and systems integrity test |
| | SAE J3058 | Storage device integrity test |
| | SAE J3059 | Measurement of EMS practitioner head movement during a crash event |
| | SAE J3102 | Patient cot subfloor integrity test |

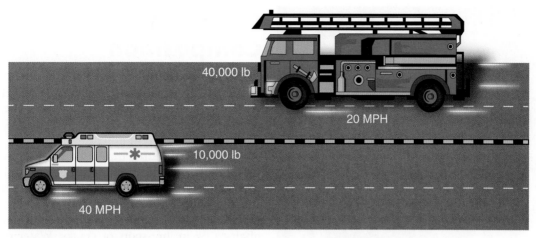

**Figure 5-6** A 40,000-pound fire truck traveling at 20 mph has the same kinetic energy as a 10,000-pound ambulance traveling at 40 mph.
© Jones & Bartlett Learning

**Inertia** is a moving object's resistance to change in its direction or speed. Inertia is affected by the weight of the object and the distribution of its weight. Additionally, inertia is affected by the speed of the vehicle—the slower the vehicle is moving, the more likely it is to resist a change of direction. A vehicle has two forms of energy, potential and kinetic. **Potential energy** is the energy the vehicle is capable of exerting, measured while at rest. **Kinetic energy** is the energy a moving vehicle has based on its weight and speed of travel (**Figure 5-6**). The formula used to calculate kinetic energy (KE) is one half of the weight (or mass, *m*) multiplied by the speed (or velocity, *v*) squared. In mathematical terms, this equation is:

$$KE = \tfrac{1}{2} \, m \times v^2$$

What this formula tells us is that the speed has a much greater effect on kinetic energy than the vehicle's weight. Simply stated, doubling the vehicle's speed quadruples the kinetic energy (and its potential to cause damage if it were to collide with an object). This is why vehicle operators must be mindful of their speed. Driving slightly faster equates to a much greater stopping distance, increased difficulty in handling the vehicle, and increased impact force in the event of a collision.

# Visibility: Your Field of Vision

Ambulances typically have multiple mirrors mounted to increase the vehicle operator's field of vision around the vehicle. You should always ensure that these mirrors are properly adjusted. Also be aware that these mirrors may block the view across an intersection or roadway. Electronic mirrors, which are installed on some vehicles, make adjustment much easier for multiple drivers. Mirrors may also have a heating element to help remove snow and ice for better visibility in inclement weather.

The use of convex mirrors is necessary to visualize blind spots on the sides of the ambulance. These mirrors give a wide field of vision, but they distort objects and make them appear farther away than they are (**Figure 5-7**). As a result, convex mirrors should be used with caution in judging distance, especially when backing or changing lanes.

It is also important to keep the driver's view of the mirrors clear. As mobile data computers or terminals are installed, it is important to make sure the terminal and its mounts do not block the driver's view of any mirror. These additional items in the cab can create blind spots and decrease the driver's view if not carefully installed.

Backup cameras are very useful for visualizing total blind spots, such as areas directly behind the vehicle (**Figure 5-8**). The technology now exists for a backup camera to share a screen with a global positioning system (GPS) unit so that the camera's image is displayed when the vehicle is in reverse. Some systems allow multiple camera heads to be utilized with one screen, and the EVO can toggle back and forth between the cameras, visualizing hazards from different angles. The backup camera should never be used in lieu of a spotter, but rather in conjunction with the spotter for a more complete field of vision while backing. However, it is important to utilize safe practices when spotters are near moving vehicles. If the EVO loses sight of the spotter(s), then the vehicle should be stopped immediately until all spotters are accounted for.

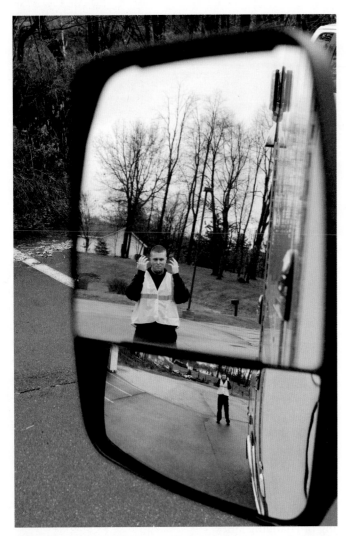

**Figure 5-7** Contrasting views from a regular mirror (top) and a convex mirror (bottom).

© Jones & Bartlett Learning. Photographed by Darren Stahlman.

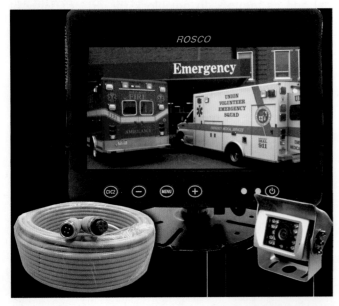

**Figure 5-8** Backup cameras increase visibility into blind spots.

© Rosco Vision Systems

# Road Construction/ Composition

To be in full control of the vehicle, you must also be aware of the driving environment. Road surfaces and shapes may affect the vehicle's traction. The main types of road surfaces are asphalt, concrete, dirt, and gravel. Each presents different potential hazards.

Asphalt is a petroleum-based product, which means that it may leech oils from its surface, resulting in a very slick surface in rainy conditions (especially when it first starts raining). In addition, asphalt repair is often accomplished by patching the surface with tar or additional asphalt to fill in low spots or cracks. Water can seep into asphalt cracks, freeze under the surface, and push up a portion of the asphalt, which results in rough roads and slick spots. When moving vehicles constantly pulverize the asphalt, potholes may result.

Concrete is typically one of the most durable road surfaces available. It is virtually incompressible, so it is commonly constructed with expansion joints, which give concrete roads a characteristic "thump, thump" feel when driving because each slab may have settled differently in places in the roadbed.

On dirt and gravel roads (discussed later), the EVO must make adjustments for the reduced amount of friction with the road surface. Stopping distances are increased on these types of roads because the surface promotes sliding between the road and the vehicle tires. In addition, like any other large, heavy vehicle, ambulances create flying bits of gravel that can be hazardous to other vehicles or pedestrians in the area and can create large dust clouds that reduce visibility. Whenever you are driving on these often-irregular road surfaces, you should be mindful of the vehicle's underbody clearance. Use caution to avoid large potholes or other irregularities that could cause the bottom of the ambulance to strike the road, causing significant damage to the vehicle.

Road shape is also an important consideration. Learning to read the road **contour** (curvature) can make you a much safer EVO. For example, noting the tree line in the distance can help alert you to upcoming curves. Roads have a **crown** (slope) to facilitate debris and water drainage from the surface. Although this is commonly a very gentle angle, on certain roadways it can relate to a large **camber** (arched surface, or road bank) and sometimes cause awkward vehicle handling (**Figure 5-9**).

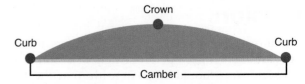

**Figure 5-9** The road's camber rises from the curb to the crown and falls back to the curb.

© Jones & Bartlett Learning

A road rises from the gutters or shoulder on one side to the crown of the road and then slopes back downward toward the shoulders/gutters on the opposite side. When a vehicle is on the road, the crown is most likely to the driver's left or just under the vehicle's left tires. The intersection of two crown roadways creates a valley at both the beginning and end of the intersection. When a vehicle travels through the intersection, its front wheels become airborne, and as they come down on the suspension, the rear wheels simultaneously become airborne. This creates a see-saw motion from front to back that becomes more pronounced as the vehicle's speed increases. If a vehicle traverses the intersection too quickly, the EVO could easily lose control.

## Unimproved Surfaces

Unimproved roads are those that are not paved, such as dirt or gravel roads. They are not limited to back roads in more rural areas and may be found in construction zones or in city parks after a heavy rain. Driving on unimproved roads raises certain considerations for the EVO.

Dry dirt roads have a loose top layer over a hard base that causes the vehicle to lose traction. Turning, cornering, and braking all become more difficult the faster the vehicle travels. Specifically, as the tires struggle to grip the loose dirt, the vehicle will tend to oversteer when turning and will travel a greater distance when braking. Further, ruts in the road can cause the bottom of the vehicle to hit the road and result in serious undercarriage damage to both the drivetrain and suspension, in addition to discomfort and exacerbated injuries for the patient during transport.

When traveling on a dry dirt road at higher speeds, the vehicle tends to kick up a cloud of dust behind it. This dust can be extremely dangerous because it creates poor visibility for other motorists or emergency vehicles. Keep the vehicle's speed down and check your mirrors often to ensure that you are not raising a cloud of dust. Communication is key when following another unit on these types of roads. Maintain radio contact in order to inform each other of potential hazards, and give instructions when needed. It is also important to increase your following distance. The combination of decreased visibility and diminished braking creates a dangerous scenario in which you have less visual notice of the need to stop, yet need a great distance to stop.

During the wet season, dirt roads become muddy roads, which can cause the vehicle to lose traction as it slides around on the slick mud. The mud may be so deep in some parts that vehicles can become stuck in a rut or mud hole and require a tow truck for assistance. Lead vehicles can potentially also throw a lot of mud out from their back tires, causing poor visibility for following vehicles.

Gravel roads have all of the issues mentioned for dirt roads plus an increased risk of kicking up stones that can damage other vehicles or injure pedestrians and bystanders. When following another vehicle on a gravel road, increase your following distance to ensure that flying stones and debris do not damage your windshield or other parts of the vehicle.

Agencies should have a standard operating procedure (SOP) in place that defines what roads, paths, or easements are permissible to drive on within their response areas. Remember that if you are in doubt about the condition of the road, stay off of it. You are of no use if your vehicle gets damaged or disabled while responding to help others. Emergency vehicles intended for use on unpaved or partly cleared roads should be specially designed to endure the rigors of that type of terrain, and the EVO should receive additional training to ensure safe vehicle operation.

> **SAFETY TIP**
>
> While driving, pay close attention to details. The reflection of light off of phone and power lines can make you aware of these overhead hazards. Dark spots in the center of the driving lane may indicate oil drops, a potential slippery hazard.

> **SAFETY TIP**
>
> Take special care on narrow roads not to drop a wheel off the road edge. If the vehicle does run off the roadway, remove your foot from the accelerator and steer it back onto the road slowly and gently as the vehicle slows down. Do not hit the brakes or turn the wheel forcefully to return the vehicle to the roadway, as doing so could lead to overcorrection and cause the vehicle to veer across the center line and possibly overturn.

## Quality of the Ride

The biggest difference in operating an ambulance versus any other road vehicle is that you are transporting sick or injured patients. The EVO must find a safe balance between rapid transport to a medical facility and smooth driving for the patient and the practitioner providing care while en route. A good EVO always considers the patient's condition; for example, a conscious patient with a painful fracture may require extreme caution while crossing railroad tracks.

Remember that ongoing patient care is being provided in the rear of the ambulance. Taking time to maneuver the vehicle for a smooth, safe ride may increase travel time slightly but reduces the likelihood of a collision and allows for easier patient care and comfort during transport. Acceleration and deceleration are felt exponentially in the back of the unit versus in the driver compartment. This means that the EVO needs to be conscious of the rate of acceleration during takeoff and deceleration during stops. The EVO should also alert the crew if there will be any sudden change in speed, roughness of ride, or direction. As discussed previously, the few seconds saved by rough, urgent transport will not likely make a difference in the patient's clinical outcome and will place everyone in the vehicle in greater, and unnecessary, danger.

---

### SAFETY TIP

Emergency transportation from the scene to the hospital should be carefully considered based on the patient's clinical condition and in accordance with local standard operating procedures (SOPs) and agency guidelines.

---

## Safety Cushion

The EVO should understand and employ a **safety cushion** around the vehicle. This entails keeping a safe **following distance** from the vehicle in front, having an awareness of other vehicles or objects to the rear, and maintaining sufficient vehicle clearance on the sides of the vehicle.

To determine the correct following distance, you should take into account the total stopping distance of the vehicle, which includes perception distance, reaction distance, and braking distance. **Perception distance** is the amount of distance the vehicle travels during the time it takes for you to recognize a particular hazard. The average person takes 0.5 to 2 seconds to decide to stop versus making another move such as a lane change. **Reaction distance** is the distance the vehicle travels during your reaction to that hazard. **Braking distance** is the physical stopping distance of the vehicle with the brakes applied. For example, suppose a vehicle in front of you is slowing down. The perception distance would be the distance traveled while you turn your eyes to the road and perceive the hazard, the reaction distance would be the distance the vehicle travels from this moment of recognition until your foot presses on the brakes, and the braking distance would be the distance traveled from the time you press on the brakes to the moment the vehicle comes to a stop. **Table 5-3** shows average distances traveled during perception and reaction time, braking distances at various speeds, and the overall stopping distances at these speeds. Remember, this table is for cars, not ambulances, which are heavier and require greater stopping distances. The table shows miles per hour as feet per second that the car is traveling.

For a general guideline, the following distance can be calculated by the **4-5-12 rule**. This rule recommends maintaining a 4-second interval between your vehicle and the vehicle ahead for speeds below 55 mph; increasing the interval to 5 seconds when traveling at speeds above 55 mph; and adding a 12-second visual lead time, which is to say that you should always be looking 12 seconds ahead for possible hazards and alternate travel paths.

| Table 5-3 Calculating Following Distance | | | | | | |
|---|---|---|---|---|---|---|
| **Miles per Hour** | **Feet per Second** | **Perception Reaction Distance (feet)** | **Braking Distance (feet)** | | **Stopping Distance (feet)** | |
| | | | Dry | Wet | Dry | Wet |
| 20 | 29 | 44 | 19 | 24 | 63 | 68 |
| 30 | 44 | 66 | 43 | 55 | 109 | 121 |
| 40 | 59 | 88 | 76 | 97 | 164 | 185 |
| 50 | 73 | 110 | 119 | 152 | 229 | 262 |
| 55 | 81 | 121 | 144 | 183 | 265 | 304 |
| 60 | 88 | 132 | 171 | 218 | 303 | 350 |
| 65 | 95 | 143 | 201 | 256 | 344 | 399 |
| 70 | 103 | 154 | 233 | 297 | 387 | 451 |
| 75 | 110 | 165 | 268 | 341 | 433 | 506 |

*Note:* These distances assume a perception time of 1.5 seconds and a level asphalt surface. Be aware that these distances will be increased for emergency vehicles due to their larger size and weight.

Reproduced from National Association of City Transportation Officials. Vehicle stopping distance and time. Published March 28, 2006. https://nacto.org/docs/usdg/vehicle_stopping_distance_and_time_upenn.pdf

In addition, you should be constantly scanning all of your mirrors and be aware of an escape route in case the vehicle in front of you stops abruptly. If you have nowhere to move to, you may need to increase the distance between you and the vehicle in front of you.

# Inclement Weather

Weather conditions such as rain, ice, snow, fog, sun, wind, and dust can change how you should maneuver your vehicle on the road. To increase safety in inclement weather, take the following steps. First, ensure maximum visibility by clearing and cleaning the headlights, windshield, and mirrors of debris. If your mirrors are equipped with heaters, activating the heaters will help keep the mirrors clear of snow, ice, and condensation. Second, check that the soles of your footwear are clear of debris. It is important to recognize that heavy rain or snow boots may reduce tactile sensation and pedal control. Third, adjust your speed and stopping distance based on the road conditions.

Any kind of wet weather demands a gentler touch with the vehicle controls. Rain and snow lower visibility and require greater stopping distances. In inclement weather, you should drive slower than usual and keep in mind that you do not have the vehicular control you would under normal road conditions. Many states have laws regarding the use of headlights and windshield wipers during inclement weather. Headlights increase visibility and allow other drivers to see you. Windshield wipers ensure that you have a clear view ahead and should be operated at high enough speeds to clear the windshield of any unexpected splashes.

> **SAFETY TIP**
>
> On some vehicles with throttle and brake side by side, there is barely a quarter inch of clearance from the brake pedal when a large boot is placed squarely on the throttle. Be careful not to allow your boots to get caught between these two pedals.

Wet weather can also affect the operation and efficiency of the vehicle's braking system. **Hydroplaning** can occur when a rolling tire rides up on a thin layer of water, thus preventing the tire tread from reaching the road surface. Most tread patterns on tires have small slits in the treads, called **sipes**, which allow water to seep up within the tread block so that the tire stays in contact with the road surface. The rotating tire sheds this water on each rotation. However, in severe wet weather or with very worn tires, the slits may not be able to empty, causing the tire to hydroplane and leading to reduced traction and directional control.

It takes only one-sixteenth of an inch of water to hydroplane. If this happens, release the throttle pedal and allow the vehicle to slow down and sink back down to the road surface to regain traction. If you start to skid, depressing the brake pedal will increase your loss of control. If the rear of the vehicle starts to move to the left or the right, slightly steer into the skid to correct the vehicle's direction. You should always operate the vehicle at a safe speed to maintain traction with the road surface. It is important to note that traction is often more reduced when it first starts to rain. This is due to the mixing of oil from vehicles seeping up from the road and forming a slippery mixture with the rain. As the rains continue, that surface emulsion is eventually washed away and traction increases. Also stay alert for any pools of water, which if contacted, can cause the vehicle to suddenly pull in that direction.

> **SAFETY TIP**
>
> As part of your routine vehicle inspection, check headlights and windshield wipers. Discovering and replacing faulty lights and wipers during the inspection is much better than having them fail when they are needed most.

One of the most hazardous winter conditions is **black ice**, a thin, clear film of water that freezes on the road. Black ice typically occurs in shaded spots or on curvy roads in areas not warmed by the sun. It may catch drivers off guard, since it is difficult to detect and the rest of the road may be thawed. Bridges and any sections of road that are open below (such as those with a large drainage pipe under the road) may also present an unanticipated hazard, as cool air may freeze that section of the road when other areas may be clear.

In general, freshly fallen and unpacked snow provides a greater degree of traction than packed snow since the tire treads are able to sink down and bite into the surface of the snow. Depending on road conditions, it may be advantageous to drive out of the ruts and onto the unpacked snow surface. Remember that ruts can pull tires in directions that you may not want to go and will probably not match the width of an ambulance. Snow can also pack up around the headlights, emergency lights, and windshield wipers, reducing their effectiveness.

Manual or automatic tire chains may be an effective tool for increasing vehicle handling on icy or snowy roads **Figure 5-10**. Automatic tire chains are controlled by the vehicle operator with a switch in the cab to allow for selective activation and are especially useful in areas where main roads are quickly cleared but rural roads may still be covered in snow and ice.

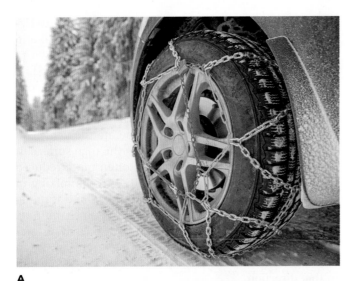

**A**

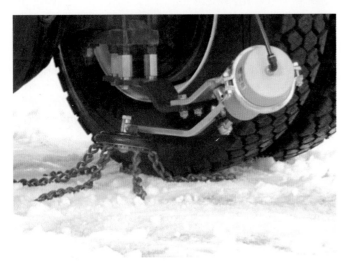

**B**

**Figure 5-10 A.** Manual tire chains. **B.** Automatic tire chains.

**A:** © Jaroslav Moravcik/Shutterstock; **B:** Courtesy of Western Bus Sales

Foggy conditions occur when moist air exists over ground that is colder than the air temperature. These areas can be unpredictable and hazardous, reducing visibility. When driving in fog, slow down and stay oriented. Depth perception and shapes may be difficult to discern, causing a delay in reaction time to any potential hazards. Consider using windshield wipers to remove the thin layer of water that can develop undetected on the windshield. Heat on external mirrors can also be useful to reduce condensation. Emergency lights should be used sparingly or not at all, as the lights reflecting off the fog may distract other motorists. In foggy conditions, use special fog or low beam headlights; high beam lights direct the light higher up, which increases the light reflection of the fog, potentially blinding the operator. Fog lights are mounted low on the vehicle and are designed with an amber lens to reduce reflectivity

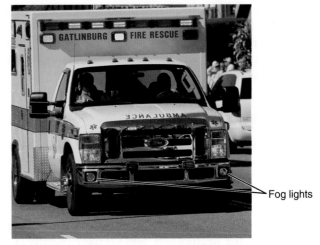

**Figure 5-11** Fog lights can increase visibility in foggy weather.

© Stania Kasula/Alamy Stock Photo

and penetrate fog (**Figure 5-11**). Also, be mindful that the effectiveness of audible warning devices can be adversely affected by fog conditions.

Wind also poses a potential weather hazard, as most emergency vehicles are not very aerodynamic. Vehicles with large, flat sides tend to catch crosswinds that can make vehicle handling difficult; slow down to reduce these effects. Headwinds and tailwinds can affect speed as well. In areas subject to high wind speeds, it is often policy to remove ambulances from service when there are sustained winds of greater than 50 mph, and to deem wind speeds of 30–50 mph as conditions that will make driving the vehicle difficult to extremely dangerous.

While not normally considered inclement weather, direct sunlight can also present a hazard by reducing vision. Use of sun visors can help. Squinting may reduce the brightness of the light but reduces your field of vision, so sunglasses are preferred. Be aware that bright sunlight can reduce your ability to see brake lights ahead, so you should increase following distances accordingly.

Finally, you may need to adjust your vehicle maneuvering to account for wet leaves and muck that can adhere to the road surface in the autumn and winter, creating an extremely slick surface at turns and intersections and potentially hiding underlying road hazards.

## Driving in Inclement Weather

Emergencies do not wait for ideal weather conditions. As such, EVOs must be prepared to work in any and all environmental situations, including dangerous weather. Following is a summary of some useful guidelines for reducing the risks inherent in driving in inclement weather.

- The first rule of safe driving in adverse weather is *slow down*! Excessive speeds are unsafe even under the best conditions, so reduce your speed to match the circumstances.
- If visibility is essentially zero (as can happen with heavy rain, fog, or dust conditions), delay leaving until conditions improve, if the call allows. If you are on the road, pull over and wait until it is safer to proceed.
- If the vehicle feels as though it is skidding or hydroplaning, do not apply the brakes. Instead, take your foot off of the accelerator and allow the vehicle to slow down naturally; this will help maintain control. Turn into the skid, not out of it.
- Fog can make it more difficult to judge speed and distance, so be sure to leave adequate stopping distance between your vehicle and the vehicle ahead of you.
- Remember that other drivers may be as unpredictable as the weather, so maintain situational awareness and drive defensively. Always know where your vehicle is in relation to other vehicles and keep an adequate amount of space between your vehicle and those around you.
- Other drivers being able to see you is as important as you being able to see other drivers. Ensure that all lights and windshield wipers are working properly when inspecting the vehicle, and when driving in rain or snow, be sure to stop in a safe location and check the headlights and tail lights for accumulated mud or snow and wipe them off them as needed. When driving in fog, use the fog/low-beam lights. Even on clear days, driving with the headlights on will make it easier for other drivers to see you.
- Wind is a particular issue for EVOs, given the design of ambulances. EVOs should remain alert and prepared to change speed and steering to compensate for gusts of wind, as they can occur rapidly and without warning. EVOs should also study their response area and determine locations with increased risks of wind, such as bridges, tunnels, and ravines. Refer to department SOPs regarding rules for operating emergency vehicles during windy conditions. Remember that large vehicles, such as buses or tractor-trailers, can also create gusts of wind as they pass, so exercise caution.

In addition, when purchasing new vehicles, agencies should consider choosing an ambulance with an **electronic stability control (ESC)** system, which is a computerized system to detect and mitigate skids. When an ESC system identifies a loss of steering control, it automatically applies the brakes, and may cut engine power, to help control and direct the vehicle. According to National Highway Traffic Safety Administration and the Insurance Institute for Highway Safety, up to one-third of fatal crashes might be prevented with this technology in place.

# Specific Vehicle Maneuvers

As an EVO, you should be familiar with how to perform the following vehicle maneuvers and understand related safety considerations.

## Braking and Stopping

In general, ambulances have a greater weight and higher center of gravity than typical motor vehicles and are therefore more susceptible to inertial forces when braking and slowing down. Slowing the vehicle can be achieved by decelerating with no braking forces (lifting your foot off of the accelerator and briefly coasting), though the operator will need to apply pressure on the brake gently as the vehicle comes to a halt to ensure a smooth and complete stop. In situations where you are cautiously allowing the vehicle to slow down but anticipate a potential hazard (e.g., if there are kids playing on the side of the street), you may choose to cover the brake pedal with your foot, but without applying pressure. This will allow a faster response if you need to apply the brakes to stop quickly.

Heavy use of the brakes can cause **brake fade**, in which the braking system overheats and reduces effectiveness of the braking system components. Brake fade is more common with heavy loads or during high-speed conditions. It is often the result of the brake shoes becoming overheated or the brake drum expanding to the point that the shoes lose contact with the drum. When brake fade occurs, braking action is ineffective and the stopping distance is increased. Some braking action may return after the system cools, but often the shoes, discs, or drums may be damaged and require repair or replacement. This is especially important for EVOs who have districts with hills and long inclines/declines. Know your district and the road hazards!

Brake fade can also be caused by two-footed driving. Having even slight pressure constantly on the brake pedal, as during two-footed driving, will cause heating of the drum and can result in decreased stopping ability and unnecessary wear on the brakes.

Some drivers mistakenly think that in order to gain maximum stopping effectiveness they can apply pressure to the brakes and skid to a halt. However, sharp pressure on the brakes can actually increase stopping distances by forming small bits of rubber that act as ball bearings on the tires and reduce the traction with the road surface. Likewise, manually pumping hard on the brakes may be ineffective because of the intermittent loss of traction (skids) caused by sharp brake application. A better way to stop the vehicle in an emergency is to squeeze the brake pedal just shy of the point of the tire skidding.

All vehicles built after 2012 have antilock brakes and hydraulic-assisted braking to aid in brake control. This requires the EVO to simply apply the brake to the degree of pressure required to stop the vehicle in a smooth,

## CRASH ANALYSIS

### Ambulance Rollover Crash with a Minivan in Intersection in Michigan

This crash involved a 2017 Ford E-450 Type III ambulance and a 2014 Dodge Grand Caravan and the subsequent rollover of the ambulance. The ambulance, crewed by an EVO and two paramedics, was transporting a cardiac patient to the hospital with lights and siren activated. The crash occurred in the early afternoon in January 2019 in an urban intersection. The roadway was straight, level, and dry as it was a clear sky with the temperature at 53°F. The posted speed limit was 50 mph; according to analysis of the event data recorder (EDR), the ambulance approached the red signal, slowed to approximately 32 mph, and began accelerating through the intersection. The Dodge had the green light and went around the right of a stopped SUV and a stopped truck with a 53-foot trailer that were both waiting for the ambulance to pass, and struck the side of the ambulance at approximately 18 mph. The ambulance rotated clockwise, tipped, and then rolled onto its left side. The ambulance EVO was a belted 44-year-old male. The rear compartment was occupied by an unbelted 45-year-old male paramedic, an unbelted 25-year-old female paramedic,

and a 79-year-old female patient restrained on the cot. The Dodge Caravan was driven by a 73-year-old female. The driver of the Dodge sustained a fractured right ankle and was transported to a local hospital where she was treated and released. The EVO complained of a headache and was transported to the emergency department (ED), treated, and released. The male paramedic sustained a concussion and chest contusion, was transported to a local hospital, treated, and released. The female paramedic sustained a fractured nose, multiple head lacerations, and forehead and shoulder contusions. She was transported to a trauma center where she was hospitalized for 2 days. The restrained patient was removed from the ambulance in cardiac arrest, a mechanical compression device was applied, and she was transported to the local ED, where she died later in the day.

1. How could this crash have been prevented?
2. Does your agency have an SOP for seatbelt use?
3. Does your agency have an SOP on negotiating intersections?

Modified from Dynamic Science. *Special Crash Investigations: Ambulance Crash Investigation; Vehicle: 2017 Ford E-450 Type III Ambulance; Location: Michigan; Crash Date: January 2019* (Report No. DOT HS 813 084). National Highway Traffic Safety Administration. November 2021. https://crashstats.nhtsa.dot.gov/Api/Public/ViewPublication/813084

controlled deceleration. When the antilock braking system (ABS) engages, you will feel a vibration or "push back" from the pedal and hear a grinding sound coming from the wheels; this is normal and you should not remove your foot from the brake because of it.

### SAFETY TIP

When stopping behind another vehicle, you should stay far enough behind so that you can see the vehicle's rear tires. This distance provides a safety cushion around the front of the vehicle and ensures that you can pull out if necessary.

Brakes are only one part of stopping. Tires must also be properly maintained because they are what actually grab the road and create traction. Rotating the tires is necessary to ensure tread wears evenly, which helps the vehicle maintain directional control. Uniform tread wear is just as important as proper tread depth when it comes to stopping. Without tires and brakes being in proper working order, controlled stopping will not happen. Vehicle and tire manufacturers provide recommendations for tire tread depth. When you see damaged, worn, or bald (low tread) tires, it is your responsibility as the EVO to contact your supervisor or maintenance team, per department SOP, to evaluate the tires.

## Negotiating Curves and Turns

Just as it does with braking and stopping, the high center of gravity in ambulances makes them susceptible to greater inertial forces when negotiating curves. According to Newton's first law of motion, an object will continue in the same direction and speed unless acted upon by an outside force. In the case of negotiating a curve, the driver steering the vehicle is the outside force and is attempting to change the direction of the vehicle. Centripetal ("center-seeking") force is also in play, pulling the vehicle inward and causing it to move in a curved path. Without this inward force, a vehicle will continue in a straight line. Friction acts as a centripetal force when negotiating a curve, and water reduces the friction between a vehicle's tires and the road surface. That is why the vehicle operator must take the same turn slower when the road is wet versus when it is dry.

Any reduction in speed by braking should be made prior to entering a curve. Continuing to brake while negotiating a curve can create problems with weight transfer. If the tires lock up in a turn, the vehicle will travel straight ahead, instead of in the direction that the wheels are turned. To safely negotiate curves, you should set an appropriate speed prior to entry, maintain steady speed throughout, and gently accelerate when exiting.

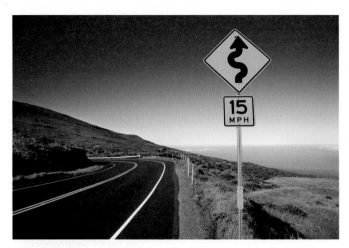

**Figure 5-12** Pay attention to curve signage.
© iofoto/Shutterstock

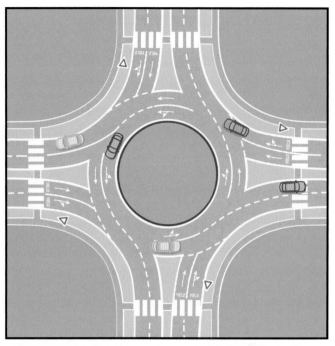

**Figure 5-13** Many communities have added roundabouts in an effort to reduce speed, yet keep the traffic moving. This is a multilane roundabout. Pay close attention to the painted arrows on the road leading into the circle.
© Jones & Bartlett Learning

When turning, a vehicle will lean toward the outside of a corner. The amount of lean, or "roll," is proportionate to the inertia of the vehicle, which is affected by the speed and radius of the corner. Typically, slower cornering results in less inertia and less vehicle roll. Similar to curves, braking should be performed before entering a corner turn to set an appropriate speed. You should negotiate the corner at a steady speed then gradually accelerate while exiting the turn.

Different types of turns may require unique maneuvering. For example, typical roads are designed so that the camber causes a vehicle to lean to the left in a left-hand curve and to lean to the right in a right-hand curve. In off-camber curves, the vehicle leans away from the curve and is at an increased risk of overturning. Similarly, turns with a decreasing radius (one in which the curve becomes tighter as it progresses) may be very dangerous. In this situation, the speed set for entering the curve may be too fast for the latter part of the curve. Operators should pay special attention to ramp warning signs and their indicated speeds (**Figure 5-12**).

## Negotiating Roundabouts

In the past two decades, there has been movement in urban, suburban, and rural areas to replace traditional intersections with single or multilane roundabouts. The modern **roundabout** (or traffic circle) is an intersection with a circular configuration that safely and efficiently moves traffic. They include curved channelized approaches that reduce vehicle speed and give the right-of-way to circulating traffic. In the United States, the traffic flows counterclockwise around a central island, usually slightly elevated, to minimize conflict points. A study conducted by the American Association of State Highway Transportation Professionals revealed an 82% reduction in fatal and injury crashes when the roundabout was compared to a two-way stop sign–controlled intersection. There was also a 78% reduction in injury and fatal crashes when the roundabout was compared to an intersection with a traffic signal. The roundabout is designed to slow speed but keep it flowing, reducing delays and queuing when compared to other intersections.

When preparing to enter a roundabout, you should first slow down. Next, you should look around at all traffic coming in your direction as well as in the direction you plan to travel in the circle. Traffic in the circle has the right of way, so be ready to yield to those motorists already moving in the circle. Often the lanes have large arrows painted on them leading up to the roundabout, which can be helpful as long as they can be seen and interpreted early (**Figure 5-13**). Note that lane changes are not permitted once in the circle, so be sure to plan your route before you enter the roundabout.

As an EVO it is your responsibility to be familiar with how to safely negotiate the roundabouts in both emergency and nonemergency response modes. While you should always refer to your state's traffic laws, the basic rules include the following:

- Remember to slow when approaching.
- Follow the lane arrows.
- The flow is counterclockwise.
- Yield to the circulating traffic.

It would also be helpful to work with the police and fire department on the traffic incident management (TIM) plan for roundabouts in your district.

## Negotiating Intersections

Extreme caution should be exercised at all intersections, since this is where the most severe crashes occur. As a general rule, you should proceed as follows. First, check traffic to the left, since this traffic is closer and presents the most immediate threat. Be especially careful at blind intersections where your vision of oncoming traffic may be obstructed. Vehicle warning lights placed on the front corners of fenders may provide an early warning to crossing traffic.

If you are crossing an intersection with a traffic light, consider whether the light is fresh (recently changed to green) or stale (a light that has been green for a while). If the green light is fresh, you may wish to wait a moment before proceeding in case any late traffic entered the intersection from an opposing direction. When the green light is stale, you may not be able to anticipate when it will change to yellow. Therefore, you should determine a braking point at which you will have to make a decision to proceed through a yellow light or stop. If there is a significant amount of cross traffic waiting to proceed, this may be an indication that the light has not turned green recently.

When it is necessary to cross an intersection against a red light, you should first come to a *complete stop* at the limit line. Once you have determined that it is safe to proceed, you may approach each lane one at a time, clearing each lane individually as the intersection is crossed. Be careful not to force stopped vehicles into controlled intersections against opposing traffic. Left turns expose the vehicle to cross traffic for a greater time than right-hand turns do. When possible, position the vehicle in the closest lane available after the turn, and then complete a lane change if necessary. This approach avoids long sweeping turns where the vehicle crosses several lanes at once. It should be noted that due to the array of warning lights on the emergency vehicle, turn signals might be washed out during an emergency response. However, you should still signal your intentions. It may seem to be helpful at times to use arm signals to traverse across traffic; however, in an emergency situation, you should keep both hands on the wheel.

Agencies should have SOPs in place to address common traffic dangers, as well as how to handle situations in which the EVO does not follow traffic laws. For example, both the EVO and their partner should submit an incident report if the EVO proceeds past a traffic control device in which they do not have the right of way without coming to a complete stop. Tracking justifications for such behavior can help agencies ensure that EVOs understand all applicable rules and regulations and help develop additional training that may be needed.

A detailed discussion of negotiating intersections safely and preventing collisions appears in Chapter 7.

## Changing Lanes

Lane changes can be safely negotiated using the mnemonic **MOST**, which stands for:

- Mirror: Look for any obstructions in the mirrors.
- Over the shoulder: Look over the shoulder when applicable.
- Signal: Use your turning signals to alert others to your intentions.
- Turn: Safely negotiate the turn.

Following this procedure ensures that the area you wish to occupy in the lane is clear.

Special care should be taken when you are passing a vehicle on a two-lane road, as you will be crossing the center dotted line (not solid line) and traveling against traffic for a brief time. If it is necessary for the vehicle in front of you to pull off onto the shoulder of the road to allow your emergency vehicle to pass, you should ensure that it has a safe place to do so and that you can safely move around the yielding vehicle with an adequate field of vision. If there is nowhere for the vehicle to safely yield, do not force it to do so. Instead, keep a steady pace in the direction of travel and pass the vehicle when it becomes safe to do so.

You should be especially cautious when it is necessary to travel in an opposing lane to pass several vehicles. Be alert for any turning vehicles occupying this lane or any "leapfrog" passers (those who attempt to pass the yielding vehicles; see **Figure 5-14**). Pass safely by indicating

> ### SAFETY TIP
>
> Most state laws require motorists to yield to the right upon approach of an emergency vehicle, so you should always attempt to pass on the left when it is safe to do so. Many larger states such as California, Florida, and Texas have changed their laws to require motorists to move to the closest curb to correspond with multilane roads. Always follow your state's specific laws!

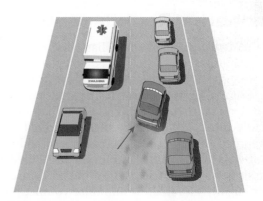

**Figure 5-14** Leapfrog passers (arrow) make for hazardous driving conditions.
© Jones & Bartlett Learning

your intent by operating the emergency vehicle toward the leftmost portion of the lane. This shows intent to pass on the left and places your vehicle's headlights within view from the motorist's side and rearview mirrors. It also puts your warning lights in view for any oncoming traffic. Take care to avoid any hazards on this section of the road such as oil drip strips or taped road lines.

## Backing

Backing accounts for a significant number of emergency vehicle crashes due to the driver's reduced field of vision. To increase visibility, use a spotter and electronic aids, such as backing cameras. Spotters should stand to the left side of the vehicle and always remain in clear view of the vehicle operator. Over the years serious injuries and fatalities have occurred in fire and EMS due to vehicle/spotter incidents. If the EVO loses sight of the spotter, then the vehicle should immediately stop. If the spotter is still not visible then the EVO should put the vehicle in park, then exit the vehicle and physically locate the spotter prior to moving the vehicle again.

Hand signals should be prearranged, and you should roll down your window to hear the spotter's instructions or cautions (**Figure 5-15**). Backing to the left, or driver's side, is usually safer than backing to the right, because

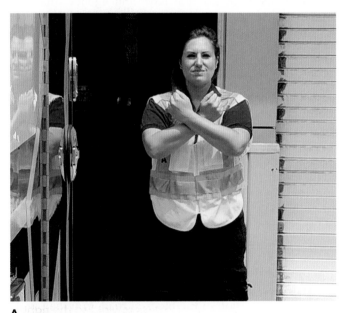

A

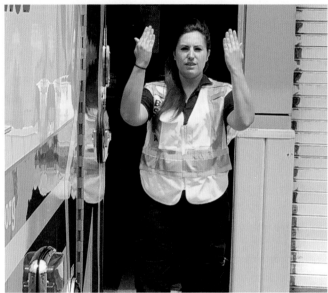

B

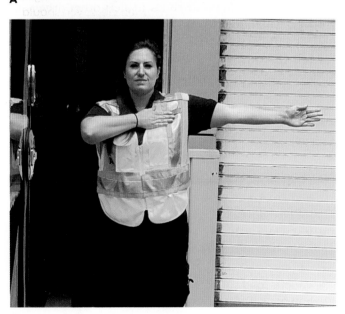

C

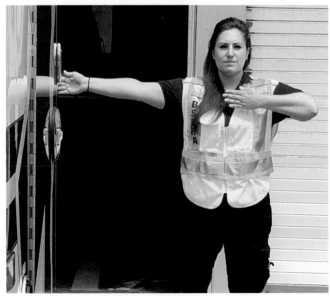

D

**Figure 5-15** Spotter hand signals: **A.** Stop. **B.** Keep going. **C.** Left. **D.** Right.

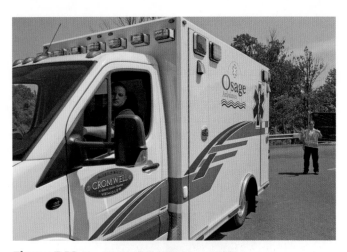

**Figure 5-16** Backing safely is a learned skill.
© Jones & Bartlett Learning. Photographed by Glen E. Ellman.

---

**SAFETY TIP**

Follow these steps for safer backing:

- Perform a complete walk-around of the vehicle to take an inventory of the area, including locating the relevant landmarks.
- Adjust mirrors properly.
- Roll window down to hear spotter.
- Use rearview camera, if available.
- Use emergency lights and back-up alarm, or use short blasts on the horn before backing.
- Back toward the left if possible.
- Position the wheels before stopping completely in the direction of your exit.
- Be aware of the location of the rear tires since they are the pivotal reference point to begin the turn.
- Remember the vehicle height when backing.

---

the operator has a clear view out of the left window. If possible, it is best to back out of the traffic flow upon arrival, to avoid backing into traffic when leaving. It is much safer to pull into traffic with the advantage of full visibility from the front of the vehicle than to monitor traffic flow when backing out. When backing into a driveway or a single lane, it is easier to back with the road to your left where you have clear vision out of the left window (**Figure 5-16**).

## Parking

Perpendicular parking is a very common maneuver required of EVOs in hospital bays and agency quarters. Perpendicular parking is usually easier if the vehicle is properly lined up with the space prior to the start of backing. This way the EVO can pick out visual cues, such as side walls or marking stripes, to assist in positioning the vehicle.

Angled parking is similar to perpendicular parking. Many parking spaces in downtown areas are angled. It may be difficult to back out of an angled space, especially into a busy road, as an ambulance has more blind spots than a personal vehicle. Some downtown spots are angled so that the vehicle operator can pull past the spot and back in at an angle, and then pull out into traffic when leaving. It is best to pay attention to the angle of the spot and the amount of room available to maneuver before determining whether it is easier to back in or out of a spot. Either way, use extreme caution when backing into or against the flow of traffic.

When parking on a hill, consider which lane of travel offers the best vision of the blocked road. You may wish to place warning flares or cones to alert other drivers to your vehicle's presence as they approach the hill. Alternatively, it may be necessary to use another emergency vehicle, such as a police car or fire truck, to block a lane of traffic to ensure safety.

---

## SUMMARY

- The U.S. General Services Administration's KKK-A-1822F identifies minimum requirements for new ambulances, provides specifications for ambulance construction, and outlines eligibility requirements for the Star of Life symbol.
- There are five different types of ambulances, based on gross vehicle weight and design.
- All vehicles have a gross vehicle weight rating that represents the manufacturer's maximum allowable weight limit of the vehicle.

- Physical factors such as friction, gravity, inertia, and energy affect a vehicle's operation and performance.
- Visibility can be increased by properly adjusting mirrors to minimize blind spots and using backup cameras and spotters.
- Various road surfaces (e.g., asphalt, concrete, dirt, and gravel) and road shape or contour may affect the vehicle's traction.

- Always remember that a smooth ride is important when transporting patients.
- An adequate safety cushion around the vehicle is essential, including a properly calculated following distance between your vehicle and the vehicle ahead of you.
- Use extra caution when driving in inclement weather conditions such as rain, ice, snow, fog, dust, and wind.
- You should be familiar with your vehicle and how to safely decrease speed and come to a complete stop.
- When negotiating curves and turns, set an appropriate speed prior to entry, maintain a steady speed throughout, and gently accelerate when exiting.
- Use the MOST mnemonic to help you remember how to change lanes: mirror check, over your shoulder, signal your intentions, and turn safely.
- Become familiar with safely negotiating a roundabout (slow down, counterclockwise flow, yield to the circulating vehicles).
- When necessary to back the vehicle, use a spotter and back to the left, if possible.
- Perpendicular parking is usually easier if the vehicle is properly lined up with the space prior to the start of backing.
- Use caution when proceeding through intersections to avoid collisions with traffic from opposing directions.

## GLOSSARY

**4-5-12 rule** A recommendation to maintain a 4-second interval between your vehicle and the vehicle ahead for speeds below 55 mph, increasing the following distance to 5 seconds for traveling speeds above 55 mph, and encompassing a 12-second visual lead time.

**black ice** A thin film of water frozen on the road.

**brake fade** A condition in which brakes become ineffective secondary to heat buildup in the braking system.

**braking distance** The physical stopping distance of the vehicle once the brakes are applied.

**camber** The banking of the roadway; an arched road surface.

**contour** The curvature of a roadway.

**crown** The slope of a roadway, designed to facilitate drainage of water and debris.

**electronic stability control (ESC)** Computerized system used to detect and mitigate skids. When an ESC system identifies a loss of steering control, it automatically applies the brakes, and may cut engine power, to help control and direct the vehicle.

**following distance** The distance between a vehicle and the vehicle ahead of it.

**friction** Resistance of an object to slide over another.

**gravity** A force that pulls objects toward the earth, resulting in what we know as weight.

**gross vehicle weight rating (GVWR)** The maximum allowable weight limit of a vehicle.

**hydroplaning** A driving situation in which a rolling tire rides up on a thin layer of water, preventing the tire tread from reaching the road surface.

**inertia** The resistance of an object to a change in its direction or speed.

**kinetic energy** The energy of a moving object based on weight and speed.

**MOST** Mnemonic that stands for *mirror, over (the shoulder), signal,* and *turn.* Used to remember the steps for safely changing lanes.

**payload** The total weight that a vehicle can carry within its gross vehicle weight rating.

**perception distance** The distance a vehicle traveosmls during the time it takes to recognize a hazard.

**potential energy** The energy an object possesses while at rest.

**reaction distance** The distance a vehicle travels during reaction time after perceiving a hazard but before applying the brakes.

**roundabout** An intersection with a circular configuration that safely and efficiently moves traffic.

**safety cushion** An adequate vehicle clearance around all sides of the vehicle.

**sipes** Small slits in the tire tread that allow water to seep up within the tread block.

# REFERENCES

American Association of State Highway and Transportation Officials. (2010). *The highway safety manual*. Washington, DC: Author.

City of Oregon City Police Department. (n.d.). Following to close. Retrieved from https://www.orcity.org/police/following-too-close

Department of Homeland Security, Science and Technology Directorate, First Responders Group. (2013). *A research study of ambulance operations and best practice considerations for emergency medical services personnel*. Retrieved from https://www.dhs.gov/sites/default/files/publications/Ambulance%20Driver%20%28Operator%29%20Best%20Practices%20Report.pdf

Dynamic Science, Inc. (2021). *Special Crash Investigations: Ambulance crash investigation; vehicle: 2017 Ford E-450 Type III ambulance; location: Michigan; crash date: January 2019* (Report No. DOT HS 813 084). Washington, DC: National Highway Traffic Safety Administration.

Oklahoma State Department of Health. (2016). *Emergency medical services statutes and regulations*. Retrieved from https://oklahoma.gov/content/dam/ok/en/health/health2/documents/ems-regulations-9-11-2016.pdf

Patrick, R. W. (2006). Safe intersection practices. *EMS World*. Retrieved from https://www.hmpgloballearningnetwork.com/site/emsworld/article/10322855/safe-intersection-practices

Sanddal, T., Sanddal, N., Ward, N., & Stanley, L. (2010). Ambulance vehicle operator: Driver behavior and performance checklist. Retrieved from https://nasemso.org/nasemso-document/ambulance-driver-best-practices-report/

U.S. Department of Transportation, Federal Highway Administration. (n.d.). *Roundabouts*. Retrieved from https://highways.dot.gov/safety/proven-safety-countermeasures/roundabouts

U.S. Fire Administration, Federal Emergency Management Agency. (2014). *Emergency vehicle safety initiative*. FEMA FA-336. Retrieved from https://www.usfa.fema.gov/downloads/pdf/publications/fa_336.pdf

U.S. General Services Administration. (2007). *Federal specification for the star-of-life ambulance*. KKK-A-1822F. Retrieved from https://www.ehsf.org/sites/default/files/2017-07/Federal%20Specification%20for%20the%20Star-of-Life%20Ambulance.pdf

Wind & Hurricane Impact Research Laboratory (WHIRL), Florida Institute of Technology. (2003). *Wind effects on emergency vehicles*. Melbourne, FL: Author. Retrieved from https://research.fit.edu/whirl/projects/wind-effects-on-emergency-vehicles/

# CHAPTER 6

# Mental, Emotional, and Physical Preparedness

## OBJECTIVES

**6.1** Explain the importance of mental, emotional, and physical preparedness.

**6.2** Discuss how mental preparedness, including avoiding distractions, is a key component of safe vehicle operation.

**6.3** Discuss how paying attention to detail helps ensure safe vehicle operation.

**6.4** Outline the key elements of a safety-first attitude.

**6.5** Discuss steps the emergency vehicle operator (EVO) can take to ensure emotional preparedness and reduce the effects of stress and emotion.

**6.6** Explain the importance of physical preparedness in emergency vehicle operation, including hearing and vision testing and hazards related to physical ailments, fatigue, and medication and substance use.

## SCENARIO

On a fall Sunday in Cranberry Township, Pennsylvania, the fog was so thick that it created virtual "white-out" conditions, making it nearly impossible to see the cars in front of one's vehicle or the headlights of oncoming traffic. An ambulance was transporting a 90-year-old patient for heart problems when it approached a standing red light. The EVO proceeded through the intersection with lights flashing, not engaging the siren until just 2 seconds before the ambulance broadsided a Chevy Cavalier with two occupants.

The patient, EVO, and medic in the ambulance all suffered minor injuries, while both the driver and passenger in the car were killed. The patient eventually died of a heart condition several days later, but it was not considered related to the collision. The roadway was shut down for 9 hours while police investigated the crash. Initial reports stated that the police did not know if speed played a part in the crash, but after additional investigation, they discovered that the EVO had been driving 70 mph in a 40-mph zone and had been under the influence of alcohol. The prosecutor stated that the patient's condition did not require the driver to exceed

*(continues)*

# INTRODUCTION

Every operator of an emergency vehicle is responsible for the safe operation of their vehicle as well as for the safety of the passengers, patients, and general public who might be affected by their vehicle's operation. All EVOs must be mentally, emotionally, and physically prepared every time they get behind the wheel. Mental preparedness means having a safety-first attitude and concentrating on the details of driving. Emotional preparedness includes managing stress, anxiety, and other emotions. Physical preparedness includes avoiding driving when affected by illness or injury, undergoing regular hearing and vision testing, and managing fatigue. Obviously, the use of any substance that can alter your body's ability to react quickly to an emergency should be avoided as well. A common class of substances that is often forgotten about when it comes to vehicle operation is prescription medications. The use of any medication that comes with warnings such as "may cause drowsiness," "use caution when operating heavy machinery," or "use caution when operating a motor vehicle" should be carefully considered when working as an EVO.

**SAFETY TIP**

EVOs must ensure that they are mentally, physically, and emotionally prepared to focus on the high stress environment of emergency vehicle operations. EVOs must also recognize how stressors in their personal lives can negatively affect their performance at work, and how work-related stresses can impact their personal lives. Many organizations have employee assistance programs or other confidential services to help personnel cope with professional or personal difficulties.

The National Suicide and Crisis Lifeline, accessed by dialing 988, is available 24/7 for anyone experiencing suicidal thoughts or emotional distress.

Education, training, and experience are all important aspects of being a safe EVO; however, the most important aspect of being a safe operator is a personal commitment to safety and excellence. The concepts discussed in this chapter do not exist simply for the sake of creating company standard operating procedures (SOPs). They must be embraced by the individual emergency vehicle operator. They play an integral part in ensuring the safe operation of an organization's vehicles and limiting the organization's risk.

# Mental Preparedness

As an EVO, you must stay focused solely on the task of safely operating the emergency vehicle. The key to focus is avoiding distractions such as thoughts about what is going on in your personal life or technological distractions like cell phones or mobile data terminals. Many times the EVO is doing something in addition to driving, such as receiving urgent radio traffic or transmitting on the radio. One of the most prevalent mental distractions is mentally placing oneself at the scene while still responding. It is extremely dangerous and the EVO must instead refocus their attention on the present and the driving tasks at hand. Considering questions such as, "What equipment do I need?" and "What will we find?" can help responders mentally prepare but should not take precedence over the task of arriving at the scene safely. Failure to focus on vehicle operations can have deadly consequences.

Even during "routine" assignments, EVOs must be mindful that simple conversations about "Where should I go for dinner?" or "What are you doing after work?" can lead to collisions. In the airline and helicopter air ambulance industry, all crew members are required to have a **"sterile" cockpit** during critical phases of operation. This means that during critical phases of a flight such as ground operations, departure, or arrival, crew members are permitted to discuss only issues directly related to the task being performed. This approach increases awareness and decreases errors caused by inattention due to distraction. Research has demonstrated the effectiveness of the sterile cockpit, which can be adapted for use in a variety of settings, including emergency medical services (EMS) vehicle operation. The sterile cockpit is an important concept that should be embraced to help you perform your duties safely and effectively. Complacency is one of the EMS system's worst enemies. Remember, the smallest mistakes can lead to some of the most horrific crashes.

## Avoid Technological Distractions

There are three main types of distracted driving: taking your eyes off the road, taking your hands off the wheel, and taking your mind off driving. Generally speaking, distracted driving is any activity that takes the EVO's attention away from driving. Based on a NHTSA report, a distraction-affected crash is any crash in which a driver was identified as distracted at the time of the crash. In 2020, 8% of fatal crashes, 14% of crashes involving an injury, and 13% of all police-reported motor vehicle traffic crashes were reported as distraction-affected crashes. Cellular phones, radios, and other technological devices are a major source of potential distraction for the EVO. Many EMS systems rely on cell phones as the primary form of communication between the responding vehicle and receiving hospitals. However, cell phone and radio use distract drivers and cause them to lose focus, leading to thousands of injuries and fatalities each year. When talking on a cell phone, the driver can be distracted mentally, emotionally, and physically, leading to tragic consequences. The use of cell phones by EVOs in any form while driving is neither a safe nor an accepted practice. Some local municipalities and states have created laws prohibiting cell phone use while driving, and EVOs need to be aware of and follow such laws. These laws can include prohibiting calls from supervisors, who should avoid calling crews while they are on calls *unless it is an absolute emergency*. If an EVO does use a cell phone during a response, the passenger should be the one to hold the phone to limit the likelihood of the driver becoming distracted.

The practice of texting while driving is especially unsafe and irresponsible. There is no way in which the operator of any vehicle can maintain constant visual contact with the road while texting (**Figure 6-1**). Even if you only take your eyes off the road for a fraction of a second, your vehicle is continuing to travel. At a speed of 55 mph, it will travel 60 feet in just three-quarters of a second. Studies show that texting while operating an emergency vehicle increases the likelihood of a collision by a factor of 23 because it takes the hands, eyes, and mind off of driving. Distracted driving increases the amount of time it takes the vehicle operator to react and is a leading cause of collisions (**Figure 6-2**). There is simply no excuse for it. As an EVO, you must possess a safe and positive attitude and not engage in dangerous activities. You must aim to

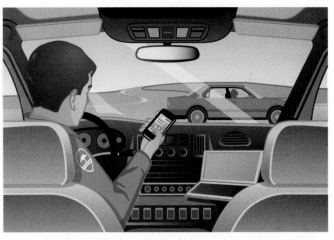

**Figure 6-1** Texting while driving puts everyone at risk.
© Jones & Bartlett Learning

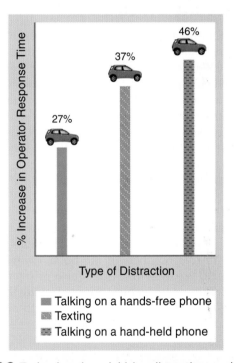

**Figure 6-2** Technology-based driving distractions and their respective percentage increase on the operator's response time.
Data from Reed N, Robbins R. The effect of text messaging on driver behaviour: a simulator study. RAC Foundation. Transport Research Laboratory. September 1, 2008. http://www.racfoundation.org

eliminate distractions and focus on the task of operating your vehicle safely. Ideally, the EVO could use their partner in the passenger seat as a "co-driver" who can handle some of the nondriving tasks such as radio use, navigation, and siren operation, as well as provide assistance with intersection clearing. Assistance with these tasks can help minimize the task saturation that EVOs experience.

Mobile data terminals (MDTs), which are common in EMS vehicles, are intended to be used only by the occupant of the passenger seat or when the vehicle is safely stopped. Use of an MDT by an EVO while the vehicle is in motion is a dangerous distraction. Operation of this type of device requires the driver to remove one hand from the steering wheel and to divert their attention from the road. Focus on the screen and/or keyboard of the device takes the driver's attention completely away from what is happening in front of and around the vehicle. It only takes a second of distraction for a collision to occur. For this reason, use of MDTs should be restricted by department SOP as well as the individual driver's conscience. "Co-drivers" in the passenger seat should be the ones to use mapping functions or MDTs whenever possible. Drivers should plan their route before leaving a scene so they won't need to look at the map while driving, unless the vehicle is stopped.

## Pay Attention to Detail

Paying attention to detail is a way of ensuring everyone's safety. As an EVO, you must ensure that everyone is properly restrained prior to moving the vehicle and during vehicle operations. You must be aware of your surroundings and environment at all times. Attend to the roadway environment and any hazards present, such as one-lane bridges, low underpasses, weight restrictions, narrow roads, or hazardous locations. Also pay close attention to your vehicle, constantly monitoring the dash, console, gauges, and warning lights. Lack of attention can create dangerous and unprofessional situations, such as driving with compartment doors unintentionally left open or partially open bay doors, leaving the garage with the shoreline still connected, driving with items or equipment left on rear bumpers or the hood, or overlooking hazards such as low wires, tree limbs, or overhangs. A quick walk around the vehicle prior to leaving the agency or scene is a good habit to avoid issues with open compartments and equipment misplacement.

> **SAFETY TIP**
>
> Adverse weather conditions can make it more difficult to identify potential hazards. When operating in adverse weather conditions, you must slow down and pay close attention to details and remain aware of your surroundings.

## Have a Safety-First Attitude

Your attitude is a key component of mental preparedness for emergency vehicle operation. Having a safety-first attitude can help you be mentally prepared. Examples of this type of attitude include remaining calm at all times,

making sure the vehicle is in safe operating condition before moving it, and constantly evaluating your driving to make sure you are doing things the safest way possible under the circumstances. Allowing yourself to be lulled into a false sense of confidence when driving with your lights and siren on can result in mistakes that can lead to a collision.

Another risky behavior is aggressive driving, which can stem from knowing that the patient is in urgent need of hospital care. Aggressive driving is not justified even in the most serious patient situations, since the time saved in transport is small, especially when compared to the increased risk of being involved in a collision. Remember that the EVO needs to keep a clear mind and focus on driving, not on patient care. Without a smooth transport, patient care can suffer. Keeping a safety-first attitude will engender good defensive driving and help combat the urge to become aggressive (**Figure 6-3**).

Having the right attitude also means not responding to other drivers who are showing signs of **road rage**. Road rage is thought to be responsible for thousands of collisions resulting in injury or death each year. As an EVO, you are held to a higher standard and should not let your emotions control your actions. In many jurisdictions EVOs are considered "professional drivers" and are held to that standard regardless of career status (volunteer versus career EMS). Do not respond to aggressors; always be courteous and remember that the vehicle you are operating is a billboard for your organization and profession. *Consider that everything you do is being filmed and could be on the Internet minutes later.* Do not take other drivers' actions personally. For example, a driver who fails to yield the right-of-way may have a vehicle with a quiet cab or may freeze when approached by an emergency vehicle. The person's response is likely accidental and they did not intend any disrespect for you or your profession.

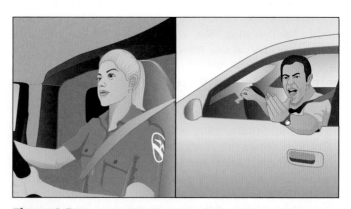

**Figure 6-3** Do not respond to aggressive drivers or let your emotions get the best of you.
© Jones & Bartlett Learning

# Emotional Preparedness

Another important factor in emergency vehicle operation is emotion. Our emotions affect us strongly and can result in dangerous behavior if not properly controlled. Negative emotions can lead to aggressive driving, while even positive emotions can be dangerous if we allow them to distract us while driving. A lack of concentration due to these very strong emotions can easily lead to a collision in which people could be hurt or even killed. Controlling emotions is a very difficult task, but it is essential to maintaining focus on the primary duty of safely operating your vehicle.

## Stress

Stress can also interfere with your ability to focus. EMS by definition is stressful, so knowing how to properly manage stressors is critical. Every person deals with stress differently, and no one technique will work for everyone. In addition, different types of calls affect responders differently. Most of us are stressed when the patient is a child, but we may just as easily be overly stressed if the patient reminds us of a loved one, such as a grandparent. The important point is to recognize when you are distressed and take action to prevent it from affecting your vehicle operation. Remember that without a smooth and safe ride, very little care will happen during transport. Furthermore, if the ambulance does not make it to the scene and then the hospital, no one will be helped.

Negative stress can cause physical symptoms such as headaches, increased blood pressure, back pain, or gastrointestinal distress. Other signs that you are stressed include rapid breathing, nervousness or shaking, and a strong urge to do everything as quickly as possible. These physical symptoms of stress can also complicate your ability to operate a vehicle. To deal with stress, you must first recognize it, and physical symptoms are sometimes the best clues.

Probably the most effective way of coping with stress for most people is to attempt conscious acts of relaxation. Deep breathing or slowly counting to 10 (or higher) before leaving the scene may allow you to reduce the stress that you may be experiencing from dealing with the patient's condition, which can help prevent the stress from affecting your driving. You may need to employ this technique prior to starting the call as well. EVOs must be able to manage whatever emotions they are experiencing, in order to provide optimum patient care.

## The Stress of Lights and Siren Responses

When responding to what sounds like a serious call, it is easy to allow your adrenaline to push you to take risks, reasoning that you have to get there as quickly as possible. Given the prevalence of concepts like the Golden Hour/ Period, which stress the need to minimize delays in delivering a critical patient to definitive care, the use of lights and siren (L&S) may seem like a reasonable approach to reduce response times. In addition, many municipal contracts with EMS agencies have a requirement for advanced life support (ALS) arrival on scene within 8 minutes, and the developers of NFPA 1710 integrated this same time frame as part of the standard. This "8-minute rule" came from a 1979 Seattle cardiac arrest study where the best survival was associated with basic life support (BLS) response within 4 minutes and ALS response within 8 minutes.

However, it is important to consider the effect that L&S use has on EVOs and other drivers, as well as examine the evidence to determine if L&S use is supported by research. As cardiac arrest comprises only 1% of EMS calls, an argument could be made that applying the 8-minute standard to all priority responses, regardless of patient presentation, is arbitrary and increases practitioner and public risk without an appreciable benefit. In addition, research by the Resuscitation Outcomes Consortium (ROC) reported no association between survival and EMS time intervals (include response and transport times), suggesting that ambulance speed is not the key component of positive patient outcomes.

Studies have shown that the use of L&S shortens response times between 1.7 and 3.6 minutes. Studies have also shown that it is associated with an increased risk of ambulance crashes and the resultant injuries and deaths in EVOs, EMS practitioners, patients, and other drivers/ pedestrians. Given the lack of evidence of benefit to the patient and the considerable evidence of the dangers of an overly rapid response, a better option would be to improve efficiency at all phases of response, such as limiting on-scene actions, to quickly assessing the patient, treating life threats, and packaging for transport; establishing SOPs regarding transport destination to ensure patients are taken to the facility that can best manage their condition; and communicating key information to emergency department staff to help them prepare for the patient's arrival. All of these would help reduce the amount of time until the patient reaches definitive care without requiring risky behavior on the part of the EVO.

Your personal attitude toward safe vehicle operations is the single most important element in reducing emergency vehicle collisions. Your ability to recognize emotional responses, manage stress, and remain focused can save your life, and the lives of your partner(s), patient(s), and the public.

# Physical Preparedness

Physical preparedness is essential to the operation of an emergency vehicle. To be prepared physically, you must start by having regular physical exams, including hearing and vision tests. You must also be aware of any physical ailments you might have that could affect your driving, and you must make sure you are getting an adequate amount of sleep. Finally, avoiding any substances, especially drugs (even over-the-counter ones) and alcohol, that can affect your body's ability to function is critical. The EVO needs to be in sufficient physical shape to operate the vehicle and keep the crew safe at all times. Remember, your job is one of the most important. Every person in the ambulance depends on you. Their lives are in your hands.

## Hearing Testing

People often take their sense of hearing for granted and do things that can diminish their ability to hear, such as listening to loud music. However, as an EVO, hearing is essential to ensuring your safety on the job. Your hearing can be compromised by colds, sinus problems, headaches, and exposure to loud noises, such as sirens and air horns. You need to recognize and be honest with yourself when these types of issues are affecting your ability to hear well.

Hearing loss is usually gradual and often difficult for people to recognize until it becomes severe. Unfortunately, hearing loss is permanent, so early intervention is critical to prevent further loss. You should have your hearing checked annually to ensure that you have not unknowingly sustained hearing damage (**Figure 6-4**). As mentioned, exposure to noises such as sirens can result in hearing loss, especially when the exposure occurs over time, as is sure to be the case for EMS professionals. Noise levels within the cab of an ambulance are of particular concern to EVOs. Headsets may be needed to help keep noise exposure within Occupational Safety and Health Administration (OSHA) recommendations, which can be found in OSHA's General Industry Standards, Occupational Noise Exposure guideline (29 CFR 1910.95). The EVO needs to ensure that noise levels and use of headsets

do not interfere with their ability to hear other emergency vehicles or outside warning devices and should consider a hearing conservation program as outlined in OSHA 29 CFR 1910.95(c).

If an EVO has hearing loss, hearing aids may provide great assistance. Hearing aids must be worn correctly, with the volume properly adjusted.

**SAFETY TIP**

Use of the siren and other audible warning devices may affect the EVO's hearing over time, thereby increasing the risk of vehicle collisions. EMS leaders and personnel should ensure systems are in place to measure and prevent hearing loss, such as requiring regular hearing tests. The siren speaker should not be mounted directly over the front cab, and vehicle windows should be closed to minimize siren noise in the cab. Some services have also considered the use of ear protection.

## Vision Testing

While it may seem obvious that a person should have good vision to safely operate an emergency vehicle, there are many people who drive every day with serious visual impairments. There are many conditions that can affect a person's vision, including the following:

- Color blindness
- Night blindness
- Farsightedness (hyperopia)
- Nearsightedness (myopia)
- Eye irritation
- Age-related vision changes
- Medical conditions (e.g., colds or allergies)
- Incorrect eyeglass or contact lens prescriptions
- Self-tinting eyeglass lenses
- Failure to get annual eye exams

It is important to recognize that vision changes. Annual eye exams are necessary to pick up on any changes in vision (**Figure 6-5**). Some insurance policies cover the cost of annual eye exams, but they are necessary even if not covered by insurance. In addition, age plays a major role in your vision. It is quite common for a person to have a change in vision around 40 years of age. It is not adequate to rely solely on the eye exam given every several years to renew your driver's license as proof that your vision is acceptable. It is important to remember that if your driver's license says you are to wear corrective lenses, then they are required while operating the ambulance.

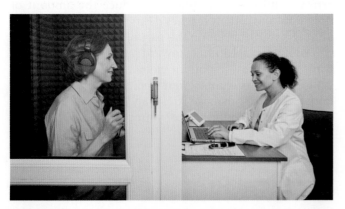

**Figure 6-4** Annual hearing tests are essential to ensure your ability to perform your job safely.
© Peakstock/Shutterstock

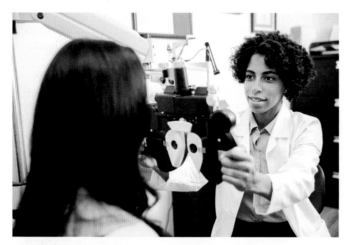

**Figure 6-5** You should get your vision checked every year.
© AMR Image/E+/Getty Images

---

**SAFETY TIP**

Some EVOs wear contact lenses during the day and resort to glasses for calls during the night. This is fine, as long as they have the most up-to-date prescription.

---

# Physical Ailments

You must be aware of your body and sensitive to any health problems, injuries, or illnesses. While many people do not think that muscle strains affect their ability to operate a vehicle, these simple physical injuries can have a major impact on your ability to function. A muscle strain can significantly reduce your ability to move your feet, legs, hands, and arms, thus increasing the time it takes you to make sudden motions. In many cases, you will not realize how much your reaction time has been affected, and when an incident occurs that requires your quick reaction, you may not be able to react to avoid a collision.

In addition to muscle injuries, a person can be injured in a manner such that they are required to wear a walking cast or a joint immobilizer. These devices are designed to help a person heal by reducing the function of the injured area. The subsequent reduction in function places the individual in an unfit, and therefore unsafe, state to operate an emergency vehicle. When a person is required to wear any type of immobilizing device, they should not operate an emergency vehicle.

## CRASH ANALYSIS
### Ambulance Driven off Road in Georgia

This crash involved a single-vehicle run-off-road crash of a 2016 Ford E-350 Type III ambulance that resulted in the fatality of a 55-year-old male patient who was being transported in a nonemergency mode. A belted 21-year-old female driver operated the ambulance at the time of the crash, with the patient and an unbelted 29-year-old male emergency medical technician (EMT) in the patient compartment. The crash occurred on a four-lane roadway during overnight hours with clear skies and a temperature of 71°F. The posted speed limit was 45 mph and the analysis from the event data recorder (EDR) showed the ambulance was traveling approximately 65 mph at time of the crash. The vehicle drifted to the right over rumble strips and departed the roadway without input from the driver. The EVO stated to the police that she had fallen asleep, which resulted in the right roadside departure of the ambulance. The vehicle then struck a large tree on the roadside, rotated clockwise, and rolled three quarter-turns before coming to rest on its right side. The patient, who was being transported on a specialty bariatric stretcher from a nursing facility to a local hospital, was displaced from the cot during the crash and suffered traumatic head injuries that resulted in his death at the crash site. The EVO and EMT were transported by other ambulances to a local hospital for treatment. The EVO was admitted for several fractures, while the EMT was treated for his injuries and released.

The ambulance service did not provide access for investigators to interview the employees, citing pending criminal and civil legal concerns. The agency performs emergency response, mutual aid, interfacility transfers, private requests, and specialty transports over multiple response areas in Georgia and Tennessee. They did release a media press release stating that all drivers were required to complete 8 hours of emergency vehicle operations training, be supervised in the field for 48 hours, and be recertified every year.

1. How could this crash have been prevented?
2. Does your agency have an SOP for seatbelt use?
3. Does your agency have an SOP on preventing fatigue?

Data from Crash Research & Analysis, Inc. *Special Crash Investigations: On-Site Ambulance Crash Investigation; Vehicle: 2016 Ford E-350 Type III Ambulance; Location: Georgia; Crash Date: June 2017* (Report No. DOT HS 812 857). National Highway Traffic Safety Administration. January 2020. https://crashstats.nhtsa.dot.gov/Api/Public/Publication/812857

Illnesses such as colds, flu, gastrointestinal (GI) distress, or headaches can also affect your ability to operate an emergency vehicle. While you may think you are not affected by a cold or a minor case of the flu, physical symptoms of these conditions such as runny nose, sneezing, or coughing will affect your ability to drive a vehicle safely. In addition, medications to control the associated symptoms will often make you drowsy. *If a medicine has a warning that says do not operate machinery, it would be inappropriate to take the medicine while working as the EVO.* GI distress can be serious as well, since having a sudden bout of vomiting or diarrhea while driving could easily lead to a collision by taking the driver's mind and eyes off the road. Even something as seemingly minor as a headache can be serious if it suddenly becomes worse while you are driving, especially if you are experiencing sensitivity to light.

During any illness, you may be distracted mentally and more likely to react negatively or aggressively toward other drivers. Whenever you are suffering from an illness, you must ensure that it is not severe enough to impact your ability to operate an emergency vehicle. You can greatly increase your risk when you fail to recognize that your ability to drive the ambulance is impaired.

## Fatigued Driving

Excessive **fatigue** is a common cause of driver error (**Figure 6-6**). Since EMS practitioners often work long shifts, including through the night, they often do not get the 7 to 9 hours of sleep that most adults require. While the rush of adrenaline that accompanies an emergency call may make us think we are alert, many symptoms of fatigue can occur even in these situations. Symptoms of fatigue include:

- Confusion or difficulty focusing
- Yawning or rubbing of the eyes

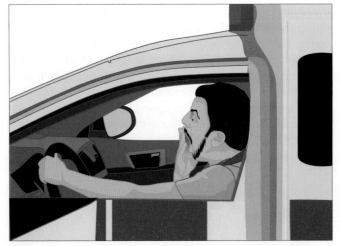

**Figure 6-6** Safe driving practices involve never driving while drowsy.

© Jones & Bartlett Learning

- Impaired reaction time, judgment, and vision
- Decreased performance, vigilance, and motivation
- Increased moodiness and aggressive behaviors
- Problems with information processing and short-term memory

Long transfers of nonemergency patients can also lead to drowsiness for the EVO and even episodes of microsleeping.

Fatigue refers to subjective physical and psychological symptoms that range from tiredness to exhaustion and interfere with a person's ability to function normally. Work-related fatigue is common in EMS, affecting more than one-half of EMS personnel, and it reduces the safety of EMS operations: Rates of injury, medical error, patient adverse events, and safety-compromising behavior are higher among fatigued EMS personnel than nonfatigued personnel.

**Microsleeping** is basically a brief lapse of consciousness or awareness that occurs when someone momentarily enters a state of sleep. A person having episodes of microsleep will experience head nodding, heavy eyelids, and periods of long blinks or seconds of the eyes being closed. Generally, microsleeping is thought to be the result of **sleep deprivation**, though microsleeping has been seen in nonsleep-deprived individuals during monotonous or boring tasks. There is little agreement on the best ways to identify and classify microsleep. In situations that demand constant alertness, such as driving a motor vehicle or working with heavy machinery, microsleeping can lead to critical mistakes—a problem that is worsened by the fact that people who experience microsleeping usually remain unaware of it.

Since the EVO is required to function with the safety of all in mind, it is essential to never drive when drowsy. Taking turns driving with your partner may be helpful, as may carrying on a conversation with your partner when you are both in the cab at the same time. If you feel you are operating the vehicle while drowsy, you should notify your partner and switch roles, if possible. If both you and your partner are extremely fatigued, you should consider notifying dispatch and asking about taking your unit out of service. The bottom line is that you are responsible for having enough sleep before coming to work that you will be able to complete your shift without encountering problems relating to sleep. Studies show that being awake for 18 consecutive hours results in impairment equal to a blood alcohol concentration of 0.05%. Being awake for a full 24 hours produces impairment similar to a 0.096% blood alcohol concentration, which is considered legally drunk in all 50 states.

While recognizing and reducing one's fatigue is ultimately the responsibility of each EMS practitioner, the EMS agency should be proactive in fatigue prevention as well. In 2013, the National EMS Advisory Council recommended the development of **evidence-based guidelines (EBGs)** for fatigue risk management tailored to EMS operations. An expert panel reviewed the available literature and produced the following five recommendations for EMS administrators:

- Use validated survey instruments to evaluate and monitor fatigue in EMS personnel.
- Reduce shift length to less than 24 hours.
- Provide caffeine to counteract the effects of fatigue.
- Allow personnel to nap while on duty to reduce fatigue.
- Provide EMS personnel with education regarding fatigue and ways to mitigate it.

Agencies should also develop SOPs to provide clear expectations regarding the risks associated with working (either as an EVO or in the patient compartment) when fatigued and outline resources available for EMS personnel to manage their fatigue.

## Shift Work and Sleep

All practitioners have their own circadian rhythms and hormones that physiologically regulate their sleep and wake cycles. EMS offers several styles of shifts, and it is important for practitioners to find the shift that best accommodates their lifestyle. For example, one practitioner was working the day shift from 7:00 AM to 7:00 PM but did not want to get up in the morning and had trouble getting to work and being prepared for calls without several cups of coffee. The same employee moved to nightshift, which was from 7:00 PM to 7:00 AM and woke up regularly without an alarm clock, was active prior to going to work, and arrived at work ready to take calls. Even when the activities were similar after work and this person stayed up until 11:00 AM on nights and 11:00 PM on days, the employee functioned better on nights than on days.

EVOs should attempt to find shifts that fit their personal rhythms and needs. In many cases, maintaining an ideal sleep schedule is not easy or possible, but doing so will help ensure that the emergency vehicle operator has the necessary energy to function properly.

## Medication or Substance Use

Occasionally, EMS practitioners will get sick, and it may be necessary to take medications that can affect their ability to perform their jobs. Before you take any over-the-counter medications, read the labels to ensure they will not compromise your ability to function, and never take any medication that warns of drowsiness and advises against operating machinery or motor vehicles. You should be aware of any potential synergistic effects with other medications or caffeine. Be sure to read and understand all warning labels and package inserts before taking any medication (**Figure 6-7**). Be especially cautious with cold, allergy, pain, diet, or sleep medications

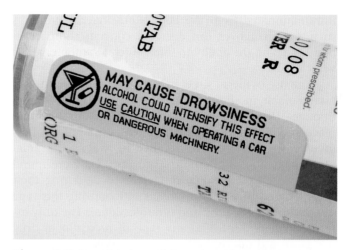

**Figure 6-7** Read labels carefully and avoid medications that can cause drowsiness.
© Wellford Tiller/Shutterstock

---

**SAFETY TIP**

*Always* read medication labels carefully and seek advice from your pharmacist prior to taking a new medication.

---

Sleep aids are available over the counter and come in many forms. Studies indicate that sleep aids can cause effects more severe than alcohol, even hours after being taken. There are documented cases of what is known as "sleep driving" in which a person gets out of bed and drives without any memory of the event. EMS practitioners should never take any form of sleep aid while at work or prior to a shift. If you are prescribed a sleep aid, you should consult your physician to determine what the time frame is between using the medication and reporting for work.

Although the use of alcohol prior to or during a shift seems ludicrous to many EMS practitioners, there are some who use alcohol and then operate emergency vehicles and provide patient care. This may seem more likely to be a problem with volunteer services, but it occurs in paid EMS services as well. This behavior is unprofessional and dangerous to everyone involved. The federal blood alcohol limit for commercial drivers is 0.04%, but EVOs follow local and state-specific regulations and are not subject to the federal transportation rules for other commercial transportation workers. Even before this level, alcohol can slow reaction time, impair vision, cause drowsiness, and impair a person's ability to function and make good decisions.

It is also important that employees are aware of, and employers have, SOPs that prohibit alcohol consumption for at least 8 hours prior to shift. These policies will help EVOs be cognizant that alcohol takes time to be fully eliminated from the body. Remember, conditions such as a hangover can decrease concentration, reaction time, and the ability to safely operate an emergency vehicle.

The use of illegal street or other recreational drugs is unacceptable in all forms and at all times by EMS practitioners. Drugs can greatly reduce your ability to think, react, and function. In some instances, EMS practitioners involved in incidents that resulted in patient and practitioner fatalities and criminal prosecutions were found to have used recreational drugs before or during their shift. Any attitude that promotes rationalizing this type of activity is unhealthy and unprofessional. The only attitude to have regarding any type of recreational drug use is an attitude of zero tolerance. With many states starting to make recreational marijuana use legal, it is important that employees and employers have clear policies addressing the use of this drug (**Figure 6-8**). As of April 2023, 38 states, three territories and the District of Columbia allow medical use of cannabis products, and as of June 2023, 23 states, two territories and the District of Columbia have enacted measures to regulate cannabis for adult nonmedical use.

It is your responsibility to be mentally, physically, and emotionally prepared every time you get behind the wheel of an emergency vehicle. You owe it to yourself, your partner, and the public.

## SAFETY TIP

It is extremely important that EMS practitioners ensure the safety of themselves, partners, patients, passengers, and the public by being aware of the signs of sleep deprivation and other detractions from their focus and awareness.

### Recreational and Medical Marijuana

Applicants for employment and volunteer opportunities should be aware of the City of Colorado Springs' current policies concerning the use of drugs or alcohol.

These policies have not been altered by Amendment 64 as it was not intended to require employers to permit marijuana use and it specifically states: "Nothing in this section is intended to require an employer to permit or accommodate the use, consumption, possession, transfer, display, transportation, sale or growing of marijuana in the workplace or to affect the ability of employers to have policies restricting the use of marijuana by employees." Colo. Const. art. XVIII, § 16(6)(a).

This language mirrors the Colorado Constitutional provision allowing medical marijuana which states: "Nothing in this section shall require any employer to accommodate the medical use of marijuana in any work place." Colo. Const. art. XVIII, § 14(10)(b).

Civilian Policy (Civilian PPM #39), Sworn Policy (Sworn PPM #35) and the Drug/Alcohol Procedures Manual outline the City's policies and remain in effect. Specifically, Drug/Alcohol

Procedures Manual, Section II, includes:

- An employee is prohibited from the unlawful manufacture, distribution, dispensing, possession or use of a Controlled Substance in the workplace or on City property.
- An employee who reports to work under the influence of or whose performance is Impaired through the use of alcohol or drugs is subject to corrective action in accordance with City policies and procedures, up to and including termination.
- Marijuana is a prohibited drug in Schedule I of the Controlled Substances Act and it remains a violation of City policy for any employee to use marijuana.

Marijuana, whether it is used medically or recreationally, remains a violation of the Federal Controlled Substances Act, 21 U.S.C. §§ 801 et seq.

**Figure 6-8** An example of a marijuana-use policy, from the Colorado Springs, Colorado, Fire Department.

## SUMMARY

- It is your responsibility to ensure you are mentally, emotionally, and physically prepared to complete all aspects of emergency vehicle operations.
- Mental preparedness includes a commitment to avoid distractions, pay attention to details, and put safety first.
- Distracted drivers pose a significant risk to other motorists.
- Emotional preparedness includes reducing stress and emotional distractions.
- The EVO must be physically capable of operating an emergency vehicle at all times.
- Get enough sleep so you are prepared to do your job without distraction.
- An individual's physical capabilities can be affected by a variety of issues, such as illness, injury, fatigue, medication, or substance use.
- It is the EVO's responsibility to know and follow their agency's SOPs on medical and recreational marijuana use.

# GLOSSARY

**evidence-based guidelines (EBGs)** Recommendations derived from the research to help define best practices and optimize decision making.

**fatigue** Refers to subjective physical and psychological symptoms that range from tiredness to exhaustion and interfere with a person's ability to function normally.

**microsleeping** A brief break with consciousness in which a person loses awareness of their surroundings and momentarily enters a state of sleep.

**road rage** Aggressive or angry behavior by a driver of a motor vehicle that may include rude gestures, verbal insults or threats, or unsafe driving.

**sleep deprivation** The state of having an insufficient amount of sleep.

**"sterile" cockpit** A concept adapted from the airline industry in which, during critical phases of an operation, personnel are permitted to discuss only issues directly related to the task being performed. This approach increases awareness and decreases errors caused by inattention due to distraction.

# REFERENCES

Eisenberg, M. S., Bergner, L., & Hallstrom, A. (1979). Cardiac resuscitation in the community. Importance of rapid provision and implications for programming planning. *Journal of the American Medical Association, 241*(18), 1905–1907.

Kane, K. (2007). Ambulance driver charged in fatal crash will be fired under zero tolerance policy. *Pittsburgh Post-Gazette.* Retrieved from http://www.post-gazette.com/local/north/2007/11/11/Ambulance-driver-charged-in-fatal-crash-will-be-fired-under-zero-tolerance-policy/stories/200711110225

Martin-Gill, C., Higgins, J. S., Van Dongen, H. P. A., Buysse, D. J., Thackery, R. W., Kupas, D. F., et al. (2018). Proposed performance measures and strategies for implementation of the fatigue risk management guidelines for Emergency Medical Services. *Prehospital Emergency Care, 22*(sup 1), 102–109.

McCallion, T. (2012). Consider the dangers of shift work: It's important to have a fatigue management plan in place. *Journal of Emergency Medical Services.* Retrieved from http://www.jems.com/article/emsinsider/consider-dangers-shift-work

National Highway Traffic Safety Administration. (2022, May). Distracted driving 2020. Retrieved from https://crashstats.nhtsa.dot.gov/Api/Public/ViewPublication/813309#:~:text=The%20number%20of%20people%20injured,in%20distraction%2Daffected%20crashes

Newgard, C. D., Schmicker, R. H., Hedges, J. R., Trickett, J. P., Davis, D. P., Bulger, E. M., et al.; Resuscitation Outcomes Consortium Investigators. (2010). Emergency medical services intervals and survival in trauma: assessment of the "golden hour" in a North American prospective cohort. *Annals of Emergency Medicine, 55*(3), 235–246.e4.

Patterson, P. D., Higgins, J. S., Lang, E. S., Runyon, M. S., Barger, L. K., Studnek, J. R., et al. (2017). Evidence-based guidelines for fatigue risk management in EMS: Formulating research questions and selecting outcomes. *Prehospital Emergency Care, 21*(2), 149–156.

Patterson, R. D., & Robinson, K. (2019, August). *Fatigue in emergency medical services systems* (DOT HS 812 767). Washington, DC: National Highway Traffic Safety Administration. Adopted from Table 6.

Patterson, P. D., Weaver, M. D., Frank, R. C., Warner, C. W., Martin-Gill, C., Guyette, F. X., et al. (2012). Association between poor sleep, fatigue, and safety outcomes in emergency medical service providers. *Prehospital Emergency Care, 16*(1), 86–97.

Ream, E., & Richardson, A. (1996). Fatigue: a concept analysis. *International Journal of Nursing Studies, 33*(5), 519–529.

Reed, N., & Robbins, R. (2008). The effect of text messaging on driver behavior: A simulator study. *Transport Research Laboratory.* Retrieved from https://www.racfoundation.org/wp-content/uploads/2017/11/texting-whilst-driving-trl-180908-report.pdf

The Cannigma. (2022). Where cannabis is legal in the United States. Retrieved from https://cannigma.com/us-states-where-cannabis-is-legal/

U.S. Department of Transportation. (2009). *Driver distraction in commercial vehicle operations.* Retrieved from https://www.fmcsa.dot.gov/sites/fmcsa.dot.gov/files/docs/DriverDistractionStudy.pdf

WPXI.com. (2007). "Two Killed in Pennsylvania Ambulance Crash." Retrieved from https://www.hmpgloballearningnetwork.com/site/emsworld/news/10339925/2-killed-pennsylvania-ambulance-crash

# CHAPTER 7

# Emergency Response

## OBJECTIVES

**7.1** Describe how to communicate with dispatch effectively and safely during an emergency response.

**7.2** Recognize the importance of route selection to a smooth and safe response.

**7.3** Describe how to use warning devices such as lights and siren appropriately.

**7.4** Demonstrate roadway command for maneuvering around traffic.

**7.5** Outline how to safely clear an intersection against a red light.

**7.6** Explain how to transport patients safely and comfortably in emergency situations.

### SCENARIO

Steve gets a call on a rainy spring day for a 4-year-old boy whose mother found him unresponsive, not breathing, and turning blue (cyanotic) near some small toys. He and his partner plan out the route, and then Steve turns on the vehicle's lights and siren and starts to head to the scene. After a few minutes, dispatch contacts the unit and tells them that the address has changed due to a poor-quality phone conversation. This means Steve has been traveling in the wrong direction for about three blocks. He turns the vehicle around and moves quickly down the block, clearing traffic to the right. As Steve approaches an intersection with a red light in his direction and traffic blocking the vehicle's path, he crosses left of center into lanes of oncoming traffic.

He looks around the intersection and identifies a truck moving toward the intersection from his left that is stopping to yield the right-of-way. He also notes a stopped car in the lane next to the truck and another car approaching from the right, both yielding the right-of-way. He determines, with his partner's help, that it is safe and proceeds through the middle of the intersection. Just as he is about to exit the intersection, an SUV cuts in front of his vehicle from the right. The ambulance strikes the vehicle, which spins around out of control and comes to rest on the other side of the intersection.

*(continues)*

**SCENARIO (CONTINUED)**

Several factors may have contributed to this collision. First, most EMS practitioners, no matter how long they have been in the field, have some anxiety when it comes to pediatric patients. It is important to pay attention to the road and not be distracted by emotions or thoughts about caring for the patient after arriving at the scene. Second, the fact that Steve had to redirect the vehicle after going the wrong direction may have increased his level of anxiety and sense of urgency, leading him to increase his driving speed. Third, Steve was too quick to determine that the intersection was safe to cross. He should have proceeded with caution through the entire intersection, constantly scanning to ensure that there were no oncoming vehicles and constantly asking for his partner's help with clearing the intersection.

1.    Do you use a global positioning system (GPS) or computer mapping device? If so, who navigates?
2.    Are there run types that create anxiety for you when they come in from dispatch?
3.    Do you trust your partner to clear intersections for you?

## INTRODUCTION

As an emergency vehicle operator, you will have to determine how to balance the need for safety and speed in responding to calls. In situations that are considered true emergencies (defined as those in which there is legitimate belief that life, limb, or property [for law enforcement and fire department response] is in danger), it may be necessary to expedite your response within your department's standard operating procedures (SOPs). You are also responsible for staying up to date on these policies as the paradigm on the appropriate use of lights and siren (L&S) is changing (per discussion in previous chapters). In emergency response situations, you will need to know how to communicate quickly and effectively with dispatch, select an appropriate route, use warning devices, and operate your vehicle safely to arrive at the scene as soon as practical.

**SAFETY TIP**

Be ready to react to other drivers, attempt to anticipate the actions of others, and identify situational hazards as they develop. Doing so will help prepare you to handle the emergency and reduce potential conflict.

# Emergency Response
## Communicating with Dispatch

When you receive information from dispatch, be sure to identify the call location, type, and response mode. This information will allow you to plan your route and determine what equipment and resources will be necessary.

Be aware that this information may not always be accurate; if the person calling EMS is distraught, lost, or confused, or has difficulty communicating, the information can be severely compromised. Whenever possible, it is best if communication between the unit and dispatch be made by another crew member, not the emergency vehicle operator (EVO). When this is not possible, the EVO should use discretion as to when it is safe to transmit information—for example, waiting until you clear the intersection or come out of the curve before transmitting may be the safest course of action. Thinking ahead about any upcoming changes in the driving environment (e.g., intersections or curves) will help you avoid a collision.

**SAFETY TIP**

You must be familiar with your agency's area, understand the address numbering system, and learn the landmarks. Be alert for any streets with similar names (i.e., Lois Court, Lois Lane, Lois Drive, Lois Point).

## Route Selection

When determining the route to respond to a call, you should consider unique situations posed by the time of day, the day of the week (i.e., weekends, weekdays, and holidays), weather, and location. For example, during early morning commutes, traffic traveling toward the center of town may be heavier than traffic moving in the opposite direction; during off-peak travel times, you may encounter road construction; and at night, you must consider loss of visibility and traffic moving at higher speeds.

It is always best to know your route before leaving the station or the scene. A short time spent planning your route before leaving may save you time and will certainly make your response safer. If you use maps for directions, then you might look at the map and plan your entire route before the vehicle ever moves; however, with mobile data terminals and GPS technology, a trip guided by your partner will be more effective. Keep in mind that GPS doesn't work well in all areas, so map reading becomes more of a necessity and is a skill that should be developed within your local agency. A lack of map reading skills can lead to collisions (driving the wrong way down a one-way street) or waste valuable response time. Making a wrong turn due to the lack of map-reading skills can send you traveling 3 minutes in the wrong direction, then having to turn around and travel back; at this point, the crew is now 6 minutes into their response and haven't progressed past the point where the mistake was made.

Even if you know your territory well, it is a good habit to look at the map or computer quickly before leaving to verify the route you have mentally prepared. If you are in unfamiliar territory (e.g., making a mutual aid response), you should be even more thorough in planning your route or use a GPS or computer mapping device. If you have a GPS device available to provide directions, take the time to enter the destination correctly before leaving or, better yet, have your partner program it. Ensure the route the device recommends is not compromised by construction, heavy traffic, or some other unforeseen local complication. Allowing the excitement of the call to lead you to leave without knowing your route will often backfire and end up costing you time in your response.

## Use of Emergency Warning Devices

Warning devices such as L&S are used to alert and inform traffic and pedestrians of an oncoming emergency vehicle in order to aid in clearing a safe path. Emergency warning devices should be used whenever you are responding to a life or limb emergency. Taking advantage of a traffic exemption, such as driving through a red light or traveling against traffic on a one-way street are examples. As a general rule, when using L&S on a response they are to be engaged at all times, not just when approaching an intersection or taking advantage of an exemption. When you use your L&S, depending on state law, you are to be given the right-of-way, but there is no guarantee that you will receive it. While you should understand how to use warning devices appropriately, you should not assume that they will be effective. Car manufacturers are competing to create a quieter interior, which means they are blocking more external sounds, including your siren. If a motorist or pedestrian does not yield the right-of-way, you don't have it, even though they are violating

the law! It is your responsibility to stay alert, observe traffic and pedestrians, and operate your vehicle appropriately. You should always drive with caution and due regard for the safety of others.

> **SAFETY TIP**
>
> No matter what type of emergency warning device is used, it is *NEVER* safe to assume that motorists and pedestrians will take notice and see or hear your vehicle approaching. At busy intersections, if possible, make eye contact with lead vehicles to assure they see you.

There are several different types of warning lights and sirens that may be used in an emergency response. Lights come in a variety of displays and colors, and sirens provide a variety of alerting sounds. Your state and local laws, as well as your company policies, will determine the type of devices required.

> **SAFETY TIP**
>
> Even with emergency warning devices activated, it is never permitted to drive around lowered railroad crossing arms or around a stopped school bus with flashing warning lights, and you should be sure all intersection lanes are clear before proceeding through all intersections.

### Lights

Emergency lights are critical for emergency responses. While sirens are important for getting the attention of drivers near your emergency vehicle, emergency lights can usually be recognized from a greater distance and allow drivers more time to adjust to your approach. There are many types of emergency lights, and each has its advantages. Understanding the applications of these lights is important to the emergency response. Types of emergency lights include the following:

- *On–off blinking red lights* are often placed on the upper corners at the front and back of the patient compartment. They are probably the oldest type of emergency lights still in use. When these lights are operating, one side will be on while the other is off, which creates an alternating blinking from right to left and vice versa, which will attract attention.

- *Light bars* contain different colors of rotating lights mounted on a bar and are usually encased in a clear hard-plastic protective covering. New models have flashing LED lights instead of rotating lights. These light bars are generally mounted on the cabs of the unit, but they may also be mounted on top of the patient compartment. The bars usually include red and white lights, although in some locations they may include blue and/or green lights as well, depending on state, local, and department SOPs.
- *Strobe lights* are generally very high-intensity lights (usually white) that flash on and off very quickly, at a rate of several times per minute. Because of the extreme brightness and the rapid rate of flashing, these lights can be seen from a significant distance, often much farther than any of the other lights. It is important to note that the strobes can be associated with causing seizures in epileptic patients and may need to be shut down when arriving on those scenes. Strobe lights should be used in conjunction with other incandescent warning lights, due to the fact that strobe lighting does not leave a lighting trail and can create a confusing setting for other motorists.

Most ambulances have a combination of these types of lights, and in many cases, they are used simultaneously. Often when arriving on scene, the EVO may choose to turn off the strobes and the light bars but leave on the red flashing lights to alert approaching traffic of the unit's presence. Some lights, especially strobes, can create vision problems at night for other traffic as well as workers operating on the scene. When driving in foggy conditions, the EVO should turn off any strobe lights because they will reflect back and effectively blind the operator at a time when good vision is critical. Each state, locality, and department will have its own rules regarding which emergency warning devices must be activated. Often, EVOs will choose to operate in emergency mode with lights only and no sirens. This is a very dangerous action that might be acceptable in a few situations, such as when traveling slowly through a subdivision very late at night when there is essentially no other traffic. The best procedure, however, is to use L&S together, which gives you the best chance of being recognized so that others will move out of your way. In fact, many states/jurisdictions require the use of an audible warning device (siren) in conjunction with lights in order to qualify for exemptions to traffic laws as an emergency vehicle.

It is also important to note that some states have opted to have a flashing blue light on the rear of the vehicle to help traffic identify the emergency vehicle from behind as they approach it. Many states have similarly adopted a yellow or amber light on the rear of the vehicle as a familiar warning to motorists. Other strategies to increase visibility include reflective paint schemes and/or chevrons on the rear of vehicles (as discussed in Chapter 8, *Crash Prevention*). For additional best practices related to use of emergency lights, see **Appendix 7-A** at the end of this chapter, which lists evidence-based recommendations for emergency lighting from the *Study of Protecting Responders on the Highways and Operation of Emergency Vehicles*.

Many states have also adopted "move-over laws" that require vehicles to move over or slow down when traveling in the lane adjacent to a stopped emergency vehicle with its emergency lights activated. It is important to be familiar with these laws and to understand that just because it is the law does not mean that all drivers will comply.

## Sirens

There are several different types of sirens and siren sounds for emergency vehicle use. All sirens must meet a federal Department of Transportation (DOT) specification of 90–120 decibels as well as any local ordinances regarding decibel levels. Common siren sounds include the following:

- A **wail** is a continuous, repeating tone that modulates from a high to a low frequency and is generally used while traveling down a road or street.
- A **Federal Q** is a well-known and distinctive type of wail siren that is trademarked by Federal Signal Corporation. Traditionally, this is a mechanical siren requiring a brake to stop, but an electronic version is now available.
- A **yelp** consists of short bursts of modulated sound; this sound is generally used to clear traffic before entering an intersection or when traffic patterns become more congested.
- A **high-low frequency siren** repeats a high tone with a quick drop to the low range. This siren is used primarily in Europe, and some states have banned this siren on vehicles and have adopted it as a civil emergency warning tone. In states where this tone can be used on vehicles, it should be used only when a change of pattern is necessary to gain the attention of another motorist.
- A **low-frequency siren** can interact with preexisting sirens, providing secondary, low-frequency duplicate tones in 8-second bursts that can shake solid materials so that motorists and pedestrians may feel the sound waves and see their effects in nearby objects such as rearview mirrors.
- A **phaser** sounds like a ray gun sound effect and may be used as an alternative to the yelp to clear traffic, but it is a deceptively useless sound given its high frequency and poor sound penetration

(discussed later). The crew inside the cab hear a loud phaser sound, while the traffic around them hears nearly nothing.

Environmental conditions can also affect the utility of different sirens. When the air is humid, lower frequency sounds travel better; conversely, higher frequencies travel better in dry air. In addition, low frequencies are better suited for highly congested areas and areas with buildings and other dense objects that do not absorb sounds.

Higher frequencies also have lower penetration (ability of sound waves travel through objects); as such, high-frequency siren tones are less able to get through the body of the vehicle and reach the driver's ears, especially when the windows are closed. This issue is amplified by the Doppler effect, which results in a perceived higher frequency of sounds moving toward a listener due to compression of the sound waves (**Figure 7-1**). Wail and yelp sirens use different frequency signals, and therefore interact with environmental factors in different ways. This is one of the reasons why it is so important to allow a siren to complete its cycle rather than "clipping" it with the manual button. When the signal is allowed to complete its cycle, it is able to travel through its entire frequency spectrum (**Figure 7-2**) and hopefully penetrate the glass of a vehicle to alert the driver of your presence. Use of a low-frequency siren in conjunction with another siren tone can also help improve sound penetration.

Sirens tend to become **omnidirectional** (projecting in all directions) when their sound waves bounce off objects such as buildings and other vehicles, thus making it difficult to determine the exact direction of the siren's location. When a **unidirectional** (projecting in one direction) warning device is needed to help motorists and pedestrians identify your vehicle's location quickly, an **air horn** may be useful. Air horns can be either electronic or pneumatic and should be used in short, intermittent bursts. When used continuously, air horns can become omnidirectional and drown out siren sounds. Excessive use of the pneumatic air horn may also decrease the effectiveness of air-assisted brake systems.

Regardless of which sound or audible warning device is used, it is important to know the limits of these devices. Most sirens are effective only 230 feet ahead of the vehicle. The faster your vehicle is traveling, the less time motorists and pedestrians have to hear and respond

### SAFETY TIP

In general, when using the yelp or phaser siren to clear traffic, you should engage the siren approximately 150 to 200 feet before the intersection. These sounds may be more effective when used in conjunction with the wail signal. No matter which siren is used, make sure to vary the sound when approaching and moving through the intersection.

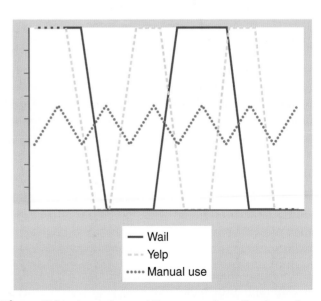

**Figure 7-1** Whether a sound is moving toward or away from a listener will change the sound's perceived frequency, known as the Doppler effect.

**Figure 7-2** When using multifrequency sirens like the wail or yelp, it is important to run the siren through its full cycle to allow it to travel through both high and low frequencies. Manually "clipping" the siren limits its range, which also limits how well the sound penetrates other vehicles.

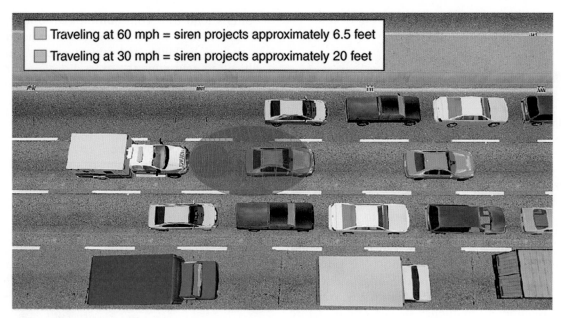

Traveling at 60 mph = siren projects approximately 6.5 feet
Traveling at 30 mph = siren projects approximately 20 feet

**Figure 7-3** At faster speeds, the siren projects a shorter distance from the vehicle.
© Jones & Bartlett Learning. Courtesy of FAAC, Inc.

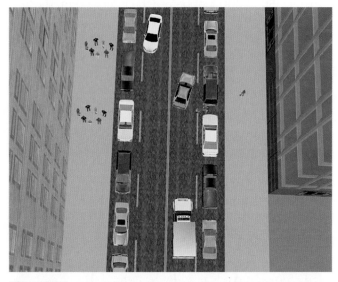

**Figure 7-4** On a multidirectional road, you should stay near the center line without crossing it to allow traffic to move safely out of the way and give you room to maneuver.
© Jones & Bartlett Learning. Courtesy of FAAC, Inc.

## Roadway Command

Vehicle placement on the roadway conveys your intentions to other motorists. When you are traveling on a multilane and bidirectional (two-way) roadway, you should position your vehicle as close to the center line as possible without crossing it (**Figure 7-4**). This allows you the most room to maneuver safely around stopped traffic. Staying close to the center line also avoids hazards such as double-parked cars, pedestrians stepping off curbs, people getting in or out of parked cars, or traffic moving to the right to yield the right-of-way.

> **SAFETY TIP**
>
> You are expected to understand basic roadway signage and striping along with traffic control devices and the laws that govern them. For a review of signage and striping, check your state department of motor vehicles (DMV) manual.

to the warning (**Figure 7-3**). If the ambulance is traveling above 40 mph, others may not hear your warning sirens in time to react; this is known as "outrunning" the siren and is a greater problem with high-frequency sirens. You should never assume that your siren will be heard by anyone, especially as car makers continue to develop quieter interiors.

When operating an emergency vehicle on a multilane unidirectional (one-way) road or those divided by medians, it is best to be in the middle lane or center of the road. This position allows traffic to pull to either the right or left to get out of the path of the emergency vehicle (**Figure 7-5**). If traffic is extremely congested and is at a standstill, traveling in the center lane will allow traffic

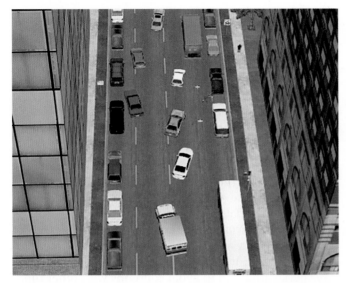

**Figure 7-5** On a unidirectional road, you can travel in the center of the road to allow traffic to move in either direction.
© Jones & Bartlett Learning. Courtesy of FAAC, Inc.

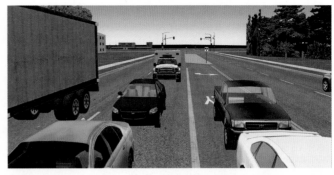

A

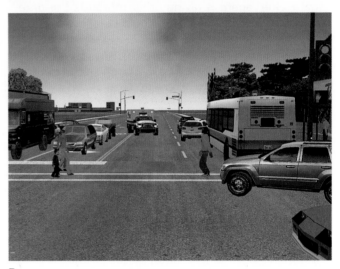

B

**Figure 7-6** Perception distance is the distance you travel when realizing that you need to brake. **A.** This distance is increased when an emergency vehicle remains in its proper travel lane. **B.** When moving left of center through an intersection, perception distance is greatly reduced.
© Jones & Bartlett Learning. Courtesy of FAAC, Inc.

to clear a path more quickly by moving into the outside lanes and shoulder of the roadway. It is important to know your state's move-over laws because some require motorists to go to the nearest curb such as on a one way street and others require them to pull to the right of their present lane.

When heavy traffic conditions will not allow you to travel with the flow of traffic, you may need to make a traffic law exemption and cross over the double yellow line into oncoming traffic. This maneuver is known as **moving left of center**. There are several important considerations you should take when moving left of center to ensure the safety of your crew and the surrounding traffic. First make sure it is acceptable by state law and company policy. It is always important to maintain a heightened level of awareness for any motorists who are not paying attention and are unaware of your vehicle's presence. Therefore, you should slow down, traveling at no more than 15 or 20 mph or slower depending on

traffic conditions, and use your turn signals to notify people of your intentions.

When driving against the direction of traffic, you should make sure that oncoming drivers are yielding the right-of-way and are moving to their right, leaving the lane closest to the center line to you. Always remain vigilant for any motorists in the left turning lane (on your right side) who may attempt to turn into your path. As soon as it is possible to do so, move back into the proper lanes of travel. If the roadway has a median, you should not attempt to cross it.

**Perception distance** is the distance the vehicle will travel while the driver is deciding on the next maneuver (**Figure 7-6**). It is shorter when moving into oncoming traffic since vehicles are approaching the emergency vehicle rather than moving away from it and the faster the vehicles are traveling, the faster the closing distance can occur. To increase perception time/distance and reduce the severity of a collision, the EVO should slow their vehicle down when traveling left of center. (It should be noted that passing another vehicle on a rural road when passing is permitted is not the same thing, and speed should be maintained so as to quickly get back to the proper lane of travel.)

---

**SAFETY TIP**

When responding with L&S, EVOs must use due regard. Due regard is giving other motorists the time needed to **recognize, process, and react** to your L&S:

- Recognize: The motorist identifies something out of the ordinary in the traffic environment.
- Process: The motorist understands the change in traffic patterns and conditions.
- React: The motorist takes the appropriate action to avoid the collision/hazard identified.

Simply entering into an intersection against the red light without stopping is not using due regard.

---

## Wake-Effect Collisions

During the response and transport phases, an EVO may be required to execute frequent lane changes and passing maneuvers. While much has been written about the risks to EVOs during an L&S response, researchers have also described a lesser-known phenomenon known as the wake-effect collisions. Wake-effect collisions are those that seem to occur as a result of the emergency vehicle passing other vehicles; they do not involve the emergency vehicle itself, but rather the other vehicles in the "wake" of the emergency vehicle. Wake-effect collisions tend to occur when:

1. The other motorists are not paying attention to their driving environment; therefore, they are not prepared to stop behind the car in front of them that has yielded the right of way to the emergency vehicle.
2. Erratic driving by the EVO and sudden maneuvers, such as sharp turns, sudden braking, or aggressive lane changes, reduce the amount of time the other motorists have to react.

Studies have shown that wake-effect collisions may occur five times more than collisions involving emergency vehicles, which is the antithesis of the most basic premise of medical care: "First, do no harm." As the EVO, it is your ultimate responsibility to ensure that you communicate your actions early and clearly enough to give ample warning to the other motorist.

---

**SAFETY TIP**

Remember that traffic law exemptions are permitted only for the time that they are necessary and when allowed by state law and department SOPs.

---

## Special Considerations

The preceding information is important on all responses, but there are other responses that will require special considerations. These include multiple-casualty incidents, hazardous materials response, and any type of technical rescue. These incidents generate a large response, with many emergency vehicles responding to the same location. EVOs need to be aware of this increased traffic and pay special attention to avoid collisions with other units. It is important to make sure intersections are clear and all vehicles are aware of which vehicles are going first and that they know not to proceed until all emergency vehicles have cleared the intersection.

It is also important to pay attention to special directions when responding to these types of incidents. Ambulances may be asked to go to a staging area away from the incident or a new location as the incident progresses. Preplanned routes may have to be adapted, and it is important that the EVO stays focused on driving and their partner in the passenger seat focuses on responding to radio traffic, navigating the ambulance, and incorporating new information as the situation develops. These new instructions could be lifesaving, especially in hazardous materials situations where chemicals may be moving.

## Intersection Analysis

One of the most dangerous maneuvers an EVO performs is crossing an intersection against the (red) light. Intersection collisions cause more damage, injuries, and fatalities than any other collision. Use extreme caution when taking advantage of this traffic law exemption. Be alert to any oncoming traffic, crossing traffic, and nearby pedestrians.

The safest way to cross an intersection against the light is as follows. Note that the steps involved are illustrated in **Figure 7-7**.

- When approaching the intersection, change the siren pattern from wail to yelp and use two short bursts followed by a pause and then two more short bursts on the air horn before approaching the intersection. The air horn produces a unidirectional sound and helps to identify your location quickly by others.
- Continuously scan the intersection in all directions and monitor radio traffic for other assignment locations in case any other emergency vehicles are approaching the same intersection.

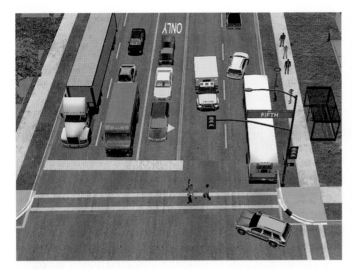

**STEP 1** Stop parallel to the rear bumper of the first vehicle in the left lane before proceeding.

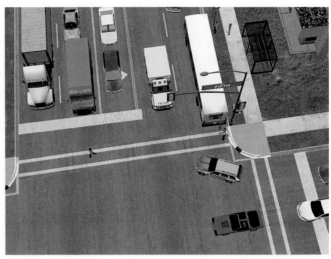

**STEP 2** Come to a complete stop at the limit line and wait for drivers to identify you.

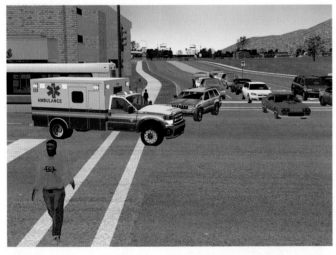

**STEP 3** Pull up to the entrance of the intersection and wait for traffic to yield.

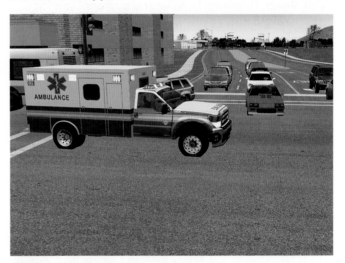

**STEP 4** Pull up to the line that marks the next lane of cross traffic and wait for traffic to yield.

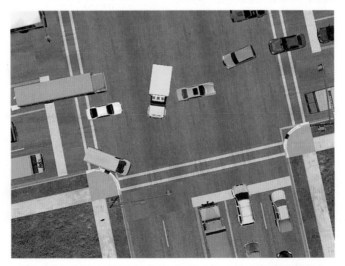

**STEP 5** Clear each lane of traffic one at a time until you are through the intersection.

**Figure 7-7** Crossing an intersection against a red light.

- Proceed slowly through the intersection. If there is other traffic waiting at the light that forces you to travel left of center, stop parallel to the rear bumper of the first vehicle in the left lane (this is to your right) before proceeding. This allows your siren to travel further into the intersection prior to your arrival and allows the driver to your right (in the left lane) to identify your vehicle in their mirror. **(STEP 1)**
- Come to complete stop at the limit line. Wait for drivers to identify you, making eye contact with the drivers if possible. Watch vehicle wheel and driver head movement to confirm that drivers are slowing and stopping, and give your siren time to travel to other motorists and pedestrians near the intersection. **(STEP 2)**
- Next, pull up to the entrance of the intersection and wait for traffic to yield. **(STEP 3)**
- Continue with the siren in yelp and with short bursts of the air horn as you pull up to the line that denotes the next lane of cross traffic. Do not pass this line until you ensure that the drivers in that lane identify you and yield the right-of-way. **(STEP 4)**

- As you approach the center of the intersection, pay attention to traffic coming from your right that may not be able to see you. Position your vehicle at an angle toward approaching traffic so that you can see the oncoming traffic and that the vehicle's **intersection marker light** can be noticed sooner.
- Clear each lane of traffic in this manner until you clear the intersection. **(STEP 5)**
- Do not stop scanning the intersection until you are completely through the intersection and traveling in your designated travel lane.

Intersections have many possible hazards, including other vehicles and objects such as buildings, trees, overgrown bushes, fences, billboards, or signs that could cause **blind spots** obstructing your view.

Blind spots can also be encountered when traveling beside other vehicles. To ensure that you are not in another vehicle's blind spot, position your vehicle so that you can see the other driver's face in their side mirror. If this is not possible (e.g., tinted windows or nighttime driving), then position your vehicle so that your front bumper is parallel to or slightly further back from the other vehicle's rear bumper (**Figure 7-8**). In this position, the other driver

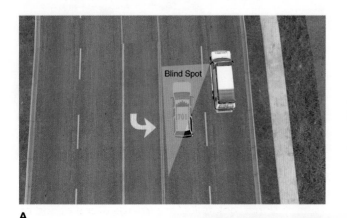
A

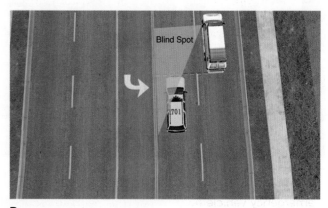
B

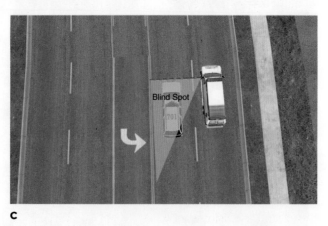
C

**Figure 7-8 A.** Do not position yourself between another vehicle's rear bumper and side mirror; this area is often in the driver's blind spot. **B.** Positioning your front bumper parallel to the other vehicle's rear bumper allows the other driver to see you in their side mirror. **C.** Parallel to the other vehicle's side mirror is also safe. When the driver looks out the window or at the side mirror, they will see your vehicle.

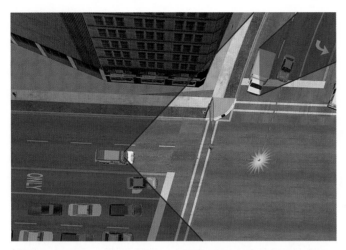

**Figure 7-9** The white truck has created a moving blind spot, hiding the green blue car so that it is outside of the EVO's field of vision.

© Jones & Bartlett Learning. Courtesy of FAAC, Inc.

should be able to identify you in their mirror. If you have sufficient room, you may also pull up, positioning your front bumper parallel to the other vehicle's side mirror so that the other driver can see you by looking out the driver's window. Other large vehicles may create moving blind spots, hiding smaller vehicles as shown in **Figure 7-9**. If the hidden vehicle accelerates, it may not become visible until the point of impact. To avoid this situation, slow down to increase your view of the situation and the amount of time you have to react to a hazard.

---

**SAFETY TIP**

An emergency vehicle preemption system allows an operator to override the normal operation of traffic lights by pausing conflicting traffic and allowing an emergency vehicle right-of-way. This helps to reduce response times and enhance traffic safety. However, a green light triggered by a preemption system can sometimes cause other motorists to take an action that can cross paths with the oncoming emergency vehicle. Therefore, the EVO should still proceed through green lights with caution, use L&S, reduce speed, and make eye contact with other drivers.

## Patient Transport

As an EVO, you will be asked to determine the need for emergency transport for patients in critical condition. You have probably seen countless movies and television shows where patients are whisked off in an ambulance with lights flashing and siren screaming. That makes for good television, but not good reality. The reality is that most

---

**OPERATOR INCIDENT**

Many intersection crashes occur every year, some with disastrous consequences. An ambulance in Eliot, Maine, was traveling through an intersection with L&S engaged when it collided with a pickup truck. While no injuries were reported, the ambulance needed to be towed and incurred $4,500 in repair costs. Two additional ambulances were needed to respond to the original call and this collision. In Portland, Oregon, an ambulance driving with L&S engaged crashed into two vehicles at an intersection. Two people were injured and needed to be transported to the hospital. The EVO was fined for failing to ensure that the intersection was clear. In Tulsa, Oklahoma, an ambulance traveling with L&S engaged collided with a car in an intersection. Again, two additional ambulances were needed for this collision and another for the original assignment. Even though most ambulance collisions thankfully do not result in serious injuries or death, they are still very costly to the service and often to the individuals involved. Last but not least, they delay response and timely care for the patient(s) involved in the original call.

---

**SAFETY TIP**

Know your vehicle's blind spots. Many ambulances have blind spots along the sides and back and below the windows and hood. The side mirrors, mobile data terminals, and A-posts (the vertical posts on either side of the vehicle's windshield that connect the roof to the body) may also create blind spots (**Figure 7-10**). Make sure to signal, look twice, and merge over a period of 10 seconds.

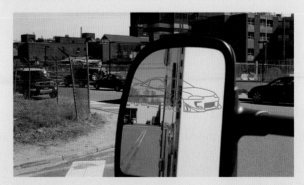

**Figure 7-10** The EVO does not see the convertible (red outline), which is in a blind spot created by the ambulance's side mirror.

© Jones & Bartlett Learning. Courtesy of Rob Raheb.

patients will not need expedited transport to the hospital with L&S, and those who do will most likely not need to travel at a speed greater than the posted speed limit.

Transport of noncritical or nonurgent patients comprises almost 80% of EMS assignments. These patients are brought to the hospital with minimal out-of-hospital interventions and will most likely be triaged at the hospital and wait for treatment. EMS crews may try justifying rushing to the hospital, claiming that speeding will save the patient's life and get the unit back into service sooner. But the truth is that treating nonurgent calls as emergencies places you, your partner, your patient, and other motorists in danger. The proper way to transport noncritical patients is to follow proper protocols: securing the patient to the stretcher or squad bench, securing all the equipment to the unit, restraining all crew and passengers, and proceeding without L&S, obeying all traffic regulations.

When a patient is in critical condition, it may be necessary to engage L&S and take advantage of traffic law exemptions. Always travel at a speed that will be safe for the patient and crew. Remember that transporting the patient to the hospital for definitive medical care is not your first priority. As the EVO, your number one job is to ensure the safety of yourself and your crew. However, bear in mind that even in the rare cases in which urgent transport is needed, you will be saving on average only about 40 seconds. If these seconds come at the price of rough handling, the crew in the back will not be able to perform the necessary patient care. Note also that in these situations equipment may need to be utilized during transport and may not be secured. This poses a dangerous condition, as the equipment can become a projectile if the ambulance takes sudden evasive action, injuring the patient or crew. If possible, vehicles should be equipped with mounts so that monitors and other equipment can be secured in a functional position.

### SAFETY TIP

The effects of a vehicle's dynamics are more magnified in the back of the ambulance than in the driver's seat. A small change in direction can throw the crew around in the back.

## SUMMARY

- As an EVO, you will need to determine how to balance the need for safety and the need for speed in responding to emergency calls.
- Communicate effectively with dispatch to gather the necessary information.
- Select an appropriate and safe route, minimizing traffic law exemptions whenever possible.
- Use warning lights and sirens appropriately to alert motorists and pedestrians of your presence.
- On a bidirectional roadway, you can clear traffic most effectively by positioning your vehicle as close to the center line as possible.
- On a unidirectional roadway, it is best to be in the middle lane or center of the road.
- When moving left of center on a bidirectional road, take the necessary precautions to ensure the safety of the crew and the surrounding traffic.
- To clear an intersection, use your sirens, scan continuously, proceed with caution, and clear only one lane of traffic at a time.
- Position yourself carefully to avoid being in other drivers' blind spots, and be aware of your vehicle's blind spots.
- Remember that you need to provide a smooth, safe ride for the patients and that a few seconds saved in transport rarely make a difference in patients' outcomes.

## GLOSSARY

**air horn** A warning device that uses compressed air, which is either electronically or manually controlled, to emit a unidirectional, long-range, low-frequency warning sound.

**blind spots** Areas that prevent the driver from seeing the path or presence of an object.

**Federal Q** A well-known and distinctive type of wail siren that is trademarked by Federal Signal Corporation.

**high-low frequency siren** A siren sound with a sharp, clipped beginning and ending that cycles through higher and lower frequencies.

**intersection marker light** The flashing emergency light on the side of the front fender, set at a 30-degree angle, that notifies motorists coming from a perpendicular direction in an intersection.

**low-frequency siren** A proprietary siren that works in conjunction with the vehicle's existing siren by producing an extremely low frequency that can shake (rumble) nearby objects.

**moving left of center** A traffic law exemption in which the emergency vehicle crosses over a dividing line and travels in opposing traffic lanes.

**omnidirectional** A sound that travels in more than one direction and can cause confusion in identifying the location of the source.

**perception distance** The distance the vehicle travels while the driver perceives a change in traffic conditions.

**phaser** A proprietary siren with a unique ray gun sound.

**recognize, process, and react** The process taken by motorists when acknowledging the presence of L&S; recognizing something out of the ordinary in the traffic environment, processing the change in traffic patterns and conditions, reacting by taking the appropriate action to avoid the collision/hazard identified.

**unidirectional** A sound that travels in one direction, aiding in identifying the location of the source.

**wail** An undulating siren sound that is effective in notifying other motorists of your presence.

**yelp** A siren sound that rises in pitch and has a short clip at the end, extremely effective for clearing intersections.

## RESOURCES

Emergency Responder Safety Institute. (2021). *Effects of emergency vehicle lighting characteristics on driver perception and behavior, study report.* Retrieved from https://www.respondersafety.com/Download.aspx?DownloadId=f31a5f73-7b95-44c7-bd25-1e4cdfce5229

Kupas, D. F., Zavadsky, M., Burton, B., Baird, S., Clawson, J. J., Decker, C., et al. (2022). Joint statement on lights & siren vehicle operations on emergency medical services responses. *Prehospital Emergency Care, 26*(3), 459–461.

## REFERENCES

Blackwell, T. H., Kline, J. A., Willis, J., & Hicks, M. (2009). Lack of association between prehospital response times and patient outcomes. *Prehospital Emergency Care, 13*, 444–450.

Clawson, J. J., Martin, R. L., Cady, G. A., & Maio, R. F. (1997). The wake effect; emergency vehicle related collisions. *Prehospital and Disaster Medicine, 12*(4), 274–277.

Cumberland Valley Volunteer Fireman's Association & Emergency Responder Safety Institute. (2018). *Study of protecting emergency responders on the highways and operation of emergency vehicles: A review of first responder agencies who have adopted emergency lighting and vehicle conspicuity technology.* Retrieved from https://www.respondersafety.com/Download.aspx?id=fa2f464f-2498-4741-917b-809592fcd789

Levick, N. (2008). *Emergency medical services: A unique transportation safety challenge.* Paper presented at the Transportation Research Board 87th annual meeting, Washington, DC.

NewsOn6.com. (2009, March 12). Tulsa EMSA ambulance involved in wreck. *NewsOn6.com.* Retrieved from http://www.newson6.com/story/9994223/tulsa-emsa-ambulance-involved-in-wreck

# Appendix 7-A. Recommendations on emergency lighting from the *Study of Protecting Emergency Responders on the Highways and Operation of Emergency Vehicles*.

- Standards-making bodies should consider reviewing standards related to emergency lighting to;
  - Incorporate research findings.
  - Take into account changes in technology like the higher intensity of LED lamps.
  - Consider new/revised requirements to incorporate technologies that have been shown to improve visibility (e.g., flash sequencing and automatic light intensity adjustment), adding maximum optical power limits to address the possible "blinding" effects of high intensity lights, and revisiting minimum optical power limits to allow for low intensity lights during night and dark operations.
- Policymakers should consider standardization of emergency lighting conventions across states, as today's mobile society means drivers are constantly crossing state lines and may not be familiar with the emergency lighting conventions in the state where they are traveling.
- Choices in emergency lighting and vehicle conspicuity should be driven by research and proven practices, not tradition and aesthetics.
- Department policy should:
  - Provide for training of personnel in emergency lighting package capabilities and usage.
  - Direct personnel to:
    - Use emergency lights to provide warning and promote move-over behavior.
    - Reduce forward-facing lights to mitigate opposite direction distractions and delays, as well as minimize potential blinding effects for oncoming motorists.
    - Display lights only on vehicles blocking traffic lanes and/or only on the rear-most vehicle when multiple responder vehicles are on the scene.
- Within the constraints of legal limitations in your state, having a lighting package that includes both use of red and blue lights is beneficial as it enables you to use red lights for daytime and low visibility conditions (e.g., smoke, fog) and blue for nighttime.
- Light intensity should be adjustable for daytime (higher power) and nighttime (lower power) conditions, preferably based on to ambient light conditions and automatically adjusted.
- Flash rates should be used thoughtfully and with regard to what research says about what they communicate to drivers. At this time, best guidance is that faster flash rates be used on vehicles in motion, as that draws more attention, and slower flash rates be used on stationary vehicles, as that helps drivers determine vehicle shape and size with less lighting distraction.
- Use emergency lighting to visually differentiate vehicles in motion (calling for right-of-way) from stationary vehicles (blocking for right-of-way). Options include flash pattern, light pattern, and light color.
- Departments should consider employing flashing light patterns of slow for stationary and fast for moving that can be automatically adjusted via a device like ambient light sensor or parking brake engagement for calling for right-of-way (faster) vs. blocking right-of-way (slower).
- Consider multilevel and high-level lighting, especially in visually dense environments like cities, to give drivers the best chance to see the vehicle and recognize it as an emergency vehicle.
- Take advantage of automatic adjustment technologies like ambient light and parking brake sensors. This enables lighting changes to happen without the need for personnel to remember to initiate them.
- White lights facing drivers should be extinguished or repositioned to point downward.

# CHAPTER 8

# Crash Prevention

## OBJECTIVES

**8.1** Discuss the factors that contribute to ambulance crashes.

**8.2** Review the importance of employing defensive driving techniques and having a safe driving attitude.

**8.3** Describe how to respond to dangerous driving conditions, such as skidding, running off the road, and tire failure.

**8.4** Outline considerations for how to position the vehicle in a safe location.

**8.5** List helpful resources for reviewing crash investigation reports.

**8.6** Identify safety technology and vehicle design elements that can help reduce the likelihood of a crash.

**8.7** Discuss what to do when a collision occurs.

**8.8** Discuss the two near-miss reporting systems and why your agency should encourage participation.

## SCENARIO

On arriving at the emergency department (ED), Mike noticed that there were several other units present and that he would have to fit the vehicle into a tight space between two other vehicles. He did not want to bother his partner, Shelly, to get out of the vehicle to assist or to look out the rear window, so he began to back the vehicle into the space to the right. Mike knew this was the worst angle, as he was reversing into his blind side, but he continued anyway. He thought he was proceeding safely and slowly, but when he impacted the ambulance behind him, the force was enough to cause his partner to fall. Shelly had been standing in the patient compartment and was placing equipment in the overhead compartment, and she fell and hit her head against the compartment door. As a result of the impact, Shelly had a small laceration to her forehead and a hematoma. A few butterfly bandages were required to close her wound, and Mike had to write an incident report.

The ambulance service investigated the incident and made several changes as a result. First, the service added language to their standard operating procedures (SOPs) requiring partners to serve as a spotter when

*(continues)*

# Ambulance Crashes: A Serious Problem

Unfortunately, ambulance crashes are relatively common, with approximately 10,000 crashes each year. One study found that from 2003 to 2007, the number of EMS deaths was 7 per 100,000 full-time equivalent EMS workers—a number almost twice the average occupational fatality rate and greater than the rate of 6.1 per 100,000 for fire personnel. Almost 60% of the EMS fatalities in that study were the result of vehicle-related incidents. From 1992 to 2011, there were an average of 4,500 ambulance crashes each year, of which an average of 29 crashes annually involved at least one fatality. These figures corresponded to an average of 33 ambulance crash fatalities each year.

There are many factors that contribute to the prevalence of crashes, including:

- Insufficient operator training
- Operator fatigue and distraction
- Driver error
- Lack of knowledge of specific traffic laws pertaining to emergency vehicle operations
- Inadequate policies and procedures for vehicle operation
- Lack of vehicle performance
- Inadequate vehicle maintenance
- Poor vehicle design
- Lack of proper safety restraints

This chapter examines steps the emergency vehicle operator (EVO) can take to avoid crashes and describes how to respond to a collision if one occurs.

# Practice Safe, Defensive Driving

William Heinrich, an American engineer, identified that for every 300 unsafe behaviors there will be 29 minor injuries and 1 fatal injury. This theory is known as Heinrich's 300-29-1 model or the accident triangle. The best ways to avoid a collision and injuries/fatalities are to limit the unsafe behaviors by driving defensively and having a safe driving attitude. This means being even-tempered, using good judgment, not demanding the right-of-way, and being courteous. Following these five common-sense rules can help reduce the likelihood of a collision:

1. Be aware of local laws and regulations that govern emergency vehicle operation.
2. Stay alert and anticipate other drivers' actions by aiming high in steering (down the road at least 12 seconds ahead) and constantly scanning to recognize any hazards.
3. Maintain proper following distance and spatial distance around the vehicle.
4. Always have an escape route.
5. Make sure other drivers can see you; keep your headlights on and avoid other vehicles' blind spots.

The EVO must always travel at a speed that is safe for the current driving conditions. Many studies have examined the time savings gained by speeding, and while the time savings may appear significant to responders, the difference is rarely clinically significant to patients. If you want to save time, drive at a safe speed along the most direct route and call ahead on the radio so the emergency department is prepared for your arrival.

Finally, to ensure safety, it is best to avoid multitasking whenever possible. During an emergency response, the EVO may be driving the vehicle, checking cross traffic, and listening to the radio or answering radio traffic at the same time. The driver's focus should be on safe operation of the vehicle. It may be necessary to delay answering a radio call until an intersection is cleared or the workload is reduced. When possible, best practice is for the EMS practitioner who is not driving to handle the radio and respond to radio traffic to minimize distractions for the EVO. The other EMS practitioners should also help clear the intersection, watch for hazards, and help navigate.

## CRASH ANALYSIS

### Fatal Ambulance Rollover in Oklahoma

This incident involved a single-vehicle crash of a 2016 Ford F-350 Type I ambulance that occurred in an interchange and the east side of a four-lane, divided interstate highway. A belted 33-year-old male drove the ambulance. An unbelted 28-year-old female paramedic and a 66-year-old female patient occupied the patient compartment. The call was a nonemergency transfer from one medical facility to another. As the highway curved to the left, the ambulance departed the right side of the roadway and struck a crash attenuator, then traversed a sloped roadside and rolled over, on its right side, multiple times. The patient compartment completely separated from the vehicle during the rollover and both the patient and paramedic were ejected. The crash occurred during the night in an area that was illuminated by artificial overhead lighting. The weather was clear visibility and cloudy with a temperature of 73°F. The posted speed limit was 60 mph and the analysis from the event data recorder (EDR) showed the ambulance was traveling approximately 88 mph at time of the crash. The cause of the roadway departure was possibly due to the EVO falling asleep. This factor was based on the paramedic's statements to the police that the EVO was unable to stay awake during the overnight shift. The driver sustained

non-incapacitating injuries, the paramedic sustained incapacitating injuries, and both were transported to the hospital. The driver was treated and released for abrasions to his scalp and extremities. The paramedic, who was found 69 feet from the ambulance, sustained facial lacerations, a dental fracture, and multiple extremity fractures. She was hospitalized for 12 days and then transferred to a skilled nursing facility for rehabilitation. The stretcher remained secured, yet the backrest broke and separated from the cot and the patient's legs slid out of the leg restraints. After the patient was ejected, she was found, still strapped to the backrest, 85 feet from the ambulance. After sustaining a large hemothorax and multiple other injuries, she was pronounced dead at the scene.

The ambulance company was involved in litigation regarding this crash, so they would not release any information regarding its policies or staff and refused requests for an interview. It was also noted at a later point that the EVO was removed from duty days prior to the crash for failing to stay awake on the job.

1. How could this crash have been prevented?
2. Does your agency have an SOP for seat belt use?
3. Does your agency have an SOP on preventing fatigue?

Modified from Indiana University Transportation Research Center. (2021, May). *Special Crash Investigations: Onsite Ambulance Crash Investigation; Vehicle: 2016 Ford F-350 Type I Ambulance; Location: Oklahoma; Crash Date: August 2017* (Report No. DOT HS 812 943). National Highway Traffic Safety Administration. May 2021. https://crashstats.nhtsa.dot.gov/Api/Public/ViewPublication/812943

### SAFETY TIP

The **SIPDE** mnemonic can help you remember the keys to defensive driving:
- **S**can: Keep your eyes moving, looking around every 2 seconds or so, and turn your head to check your surroundings directly (don't rely solely on your peripheral vision to notice potential hazards).
- **I**dentify: Recognize that a potential hazard exists (e.g., other vehicles or obstacles, road conditions, inclement weather).
- **P**redict: Based on the recognized hazards, try to anticipate possible scenarios and the actions you would take to respond to them.
- **D**ecide: Based on your predictions, choose the course(s) of action you would take if the hazard became an immediate danger.
- **E**xecute: If the potential hazard becomes an actual hazard, implement the chosen response to avoid a crash.

# Respond to Dangerous Driving Conditions

Inclement weather and hazardous driving situations such as loose gravel and leaves in the road are practically impossible to avoid; simply put, EMS cannot take time off for bad weather or road construction. Whenever possible, it is best to avoid conditions that could result in crashes, but when this isn't possible, safe vehicle operation is critical.

The most common causes of skids are driving too fast for existing conditions, failing to anticipate traffic conditions, not understanding the operational characteristics of the vehicle, misusing brakes and braking devices, and failing to properly maintain the vehicle. Some vehicles may be equipped with antilock brakes and electronic stability control to help prevent skids. In the event of a skid, you should release the brakes, allow the tires to turn to regain traction, and direct the front wheels in the direction of the skid. This means turning the vehicle into the skid and slowing without slamming on either the brakes or the accelerator.

In some hazardous situations, the vehicle may start to run off the roadway. Steering an emergency vehicle off the road can lead to a serious collision. With one wheel off the pavement, there is less traction and the driver is fooled into turning the wheel more than needed. The most common reaction is to quickly steer the vehicle back onto the roadway, but doing so may lead to a dangerous overcorrection in which the vehicle crosses over lane dividers. Instead, if you run off the road, gently remove your foot from the accelerator and continue to drive the vehicle steadily along the same path. Do not apply the brakes heavily, as doing so may cause a skid and pull you farther off the road. Gradually slow down and while keeping a firm grip on the steering wheel, smoothly turn the steering wheel to reenter the lane when traffic conditions and speed are safe to do so. It is better to strive for a slow recovery, even if the vehicle suffers minor damage as a result.

Failure of a tire, such as a blowout, should be handled in much the same way as a run-off. It is important not to hit the brakes; instead, slow to a stop and work your way to a safe place on the side of the road. The ability to steer may be greatly compromised depending on which tire is blown. Activate the appropriate warning devices to alert traffic that you are disabled on the side of the road.

# Position the Vehicle in a Safe Location

Emergency vehicles should be positioned appropriately at the emergency scene based on their function and need. For example, at an automobile crash, fire protection takes a priority, so fire apparatus must be able to stretch hose lines; if a patient is entrapped, rescue equipment must be able to reach the affected vehicle. If the ambulance is the first emergency vehicle on scene, then it will have to block the scene and should be parked with the wheels turned away from the work zone in case it is struck from behind. When blocking the collision scene, the best practice is to use "lane +1" blocking (**Figure 8-1**). Once EMS practitioners are ready to load the patient or after additional units arrive, move the ambulance downstream so that the collision scene protects the crew from traffic during patient loading. If emergency vehicles are on scene, then the ambulance should park with direct access to and from the patient, without having to expose personnel to traffic.

Ambulances should be positioned safely in a protected area at the scene. Ensure that the patient loading area is not exposed to traffic. Because most ambulances are loaded from the rear and personnel commonly operate in this immediate area, it is advisable to position the rear of the vehicle in a protected zone in front of

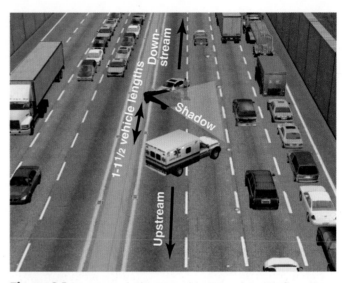

**Figure 8-1** Proper ambulance positioning when it is first on the scene or is operating alone.
© Jones & Bartlett Learning. Courtesy of FAAC, Inc.

**OPERATOR INCIDENT**

As Tim arrived at the scene of the car crash, he took the only spot he could find—in the open lane across from the damaged car—and left the vehicle to attend to the patient. Tim and his partner had difficulty getting oriented. It was nighttime and a police car with flashing lights was parked facing their vehicle, making it difficult to see. Once they found the patient and were beginning to provide care, a crewmember from a second ambulance on the scene told Tim to move their vehicle, since they had the priority patient and the ambulance was blocking the road. Tim went to move the ambulance and realized he was blocked in. After some delay, he was able to move the vehicle across the street and return to the scene. When he got back, Tim's partner told him they would need immobilization equipment, so Tim had to cross back over the busy road to retrieve the equipment.

Tim realized as he crossed the busy road for a second time that he had not considered proper vehicle positioning on the scene, and later he sought help from his training officer. The training officer advised him to consider several factors before determining where to place the vehicle, including making sure the vehicle does not constitute a hazard on the scene or block traffic, ensuring equipment is available, avoiding contaminating the area with exhaust vapors, and ensuring that crew members are not unnecessarily exposed to traffic.

the emergency scene, other rescue vehicles, and the flow of traffic. It is most effective to position the vehicle on the same side of the road as the incident if there is only partial road blockage so that personnel and preconnected hose lines are not required to cross or block lanes of traffic. Keeping one lane open will allow other emergency apparatus access into and out of the scene. Be aware of your district's traffic incident management system (TIMS) plan and follow it (TIMS is discussed in Chapter 2).

When parking at scenes where ambulances may not be needed or other vehicles keep arriving, it is important to also consider egress. At fire scenes, additional working companies and hose lines can easily block ambulances in while they are on standby. At hazardous materials scenes, it is important to make sure the ambulance will stay in the cold zone (the area most removed from exposure and with the most readily available egress) even in the event of weather changes. EVOs need to be able to take patients to the hospital. If they do not consider the expansion of the scene and always maintain a way out, they will be unable to do their job.

It is also important to be cognizant of hazards encountered at private residences and in rural areas. Many homes have low hanging power lines or outbuildings with electrical supply that some ambulances may not be able to maneuver under. Septic systems in rural yards may also be hazardous, as trucks can sink into the soft ground above the septic tank. Additionally, some homes may have privately maintained bridges that do not have posted weight limits. This presents a significant hazard for EVOs who may not know if the bridge will support the weight of an emergency vehicle.

> **SAFETY TIP**
>
> Before leaving the scene, walk around the vehicle, making sure all equipment has been retrieved from the scene and secured and all doors are closed properly. This step also provides an opportunity to observe for any potential hazards.

## Practice Safe Backing

Backing, or operating the vehicle in reverse, accounts for an estimated 25% of all emergency vehicle crashes. To help decrease the chance of a collision, a spotter should be used every time the emergency vehicle operates in reverse. As a leading cause of vehicle incidents, it is important all EVOs utilize a spotter as the standard behavior. The attitude that "it won't happen to me" is simply a justification for skipping the spotter and ultimately crashing

the vehicle. Normalization of deviance (the process of gradually accepting an incorrect behavior as correct) is a major contributor to all types of dangerous incidents, not just in regard to backing, and should be discussed with employees. This should also be emphasized in your agency's SOPs.

In addition to being a second set of eyes, the spotter is a physical deterrent to pedestrians and other motorists attempting to cross the ambulance's path. The spotter should be positioned in a safe zone on the driver's side rear of the vehicle and should be visible to the vehicle operator from their side mirror at all times. If you lose sight of your spotter in any of your mirrors, stop immediately! In situations where backing is necessary and a spotter is not available, the EVO should park the vehicle, get out, and assess the space available on all four sides of the vehicle prior to backing. Backup cameras, as well as alarms, are helpful, but a camera should never be the EVO's sole "eyes" on the situation. See Chapter 12 for considerations that agencies should follow when developing an emergency vehicle backing SOP.

## Use Vehicle Safety Technology

Newer ambulances have been designed with technology to reduce the likelihood of a crash. External cameras provide better visibility for the driver and may include multiple camera heads, allowing the operator to choose among multiple views. Black box recorders monitor vehicle operational parameters and can be used to train vehicle operators, provide information for critiques, or help in investigations. Studies have shown that these technologies can reduce the likelihood of a collision and associated damage to the vehicle or injury to the occupants. Some of these technologies will signal drivers with sounds in the cab that they are doing something potentially dangerous, while others may send real-time emails to supervisors, who can track trends in risky driving behavior.

Other vehicle design elements can increase safety as well. Adjustable seat placement and improved restraints protect attendants. Secure equipment storage can reduce risk of projectiles. (Note that cargo netting, although thought by many practitioners to reduce their likelihood of striking the bulkhead during a collision, has yet to be proven effective.) Turning and brake signal indicators in the patient compartment provide an attendant with visual warning of impending turns or stops. In addition, many manufacturers are now producing ambulances with curved and padded edges in the patient module for safety and convenience. Some are offering advanced airbag protection, along with three-point harnesses and head cushioning systems to protect attendants in the patient compartment. Seat belt monitoring devices may be installed to alert the EVO if someone in the back is not properly restrained.

Some vehicles are equipped with traction stabilization controls. Traction control is a reverse form of anti-lock brakes. In situations where one wheel loses traction (such as on slippery surfaces), torque reduction is briefly applied to slow the wheel and help the vehicle regain control.

---

**SAFETY TIP**

Even with advances in emergency vehicle design and technology, it is important to remember the most basic safety device—restraints. All occupants should be properly restrained, including those working in the patient compartment as well as any passengers and patients.

---

## Vehicle Visibility Changes

Vehicle operators may be familiar with the *Manual on Uniform Traffic Control Devices (MUTCD)* published by the Federal Highway Administration (FHWA) that defines the national standards for traffic control devices, road markings, and highway signs. This manual outlines requirements for temporary traffic controls, such as those needed when responding to a roadway incident. In addition, practitioners should be aware of the *Emergency Vehicle Visibility and Conspicuity Study* completed by the U.S. Fire Administration, which highlights best practices in emergency vehicle visibility to improve emergency vehicle and roadway operations safety. These practices include the use of retroreflective striping (a highly reflective substance that reflects light back to its source, with very little absorption or dispersion) and passive reflectors (which generally reflect light back at its source), called **chevrons**, and high-visibility paint for emergency response vehicles as shown in **Figure 8-2**. These design features are now used as a result of the study.

Research by the Emergency Responder Safety Institute has resulted in the following recommendations for improving emergency vehicle and operator **conspicuity**:

- Visibility markings should be retroreflective and in a contrasting color to the vehicle. Red and yellow or yellow-green combinations are suggested for the rear surfaces of vehicles.
- White, cream, or yellow should be used for vehicle body color.

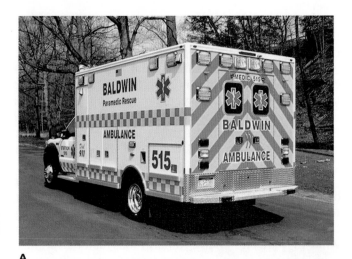

**A**

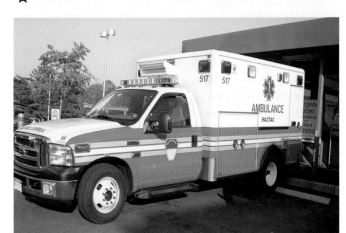

**B**

**C**

**Figure 8-2** High-visibility reflective chevron pattern on the back of an emergency vehicle **(A)**. High-visibility reflective striping on the side of an emergency vehicle in daylight **(B)** and at night **(C)**.

**A:** Courtesy of Douglas Kupas/NAEMT; **B** and **C:** © Jones & Bartlett Learning. Courtesy of Rob Raheb

- Interior surfaces of doors, tailgates, and liftgates should be marked the same as exterior surfaces, especially when opening these doors will block other warning lights or markings.
- Any attached or externally stored equipment should be marked with retroreflective material.
- When working on an emergency scene on a roadway, all personnel should be equipped with ANSI-approved high-visibility apparel.
- Ambulances should be marked in accordance with NFPA 1917, *Standard for Automotive Ambulances*, or another accepted standard.

# Crash Events

If you are involved in a crash, it is important to be familiar with state and local laws as well as the agency's SOPs. For example, many state and local laws require a motorist and vehicle involved in a collision to remain at the scene until police and/or other emergency vehicles arrive and permit them to leave. Agency SOPs may specify the following actions by the EVO:

- Report the incident via radio or per protocol.
- Secure the scene to ensure safety until law enforcement or other responders can arrive.
- Take care of any injured persons, including the EVO and other EMS personnel.
- Make no statements to anyone except law enforcement officers or your supervisors until instructed to do so by and in the presence of legal counsel. This includes social media posts!
- Fill out required reporting documents.
- Secure any equipment, such as narcotics and computers, if the unit will be towed and held for investigation.

In addition, SOPs may indicate that supervisors should photograph the scene for reports. If the involved EVO is not a supervisor, they may need to discuss the need for photographs with their supervisor.

Companies should make sure employees receive any treatment and care before paperwork is done. However, EVOs should attempt to complete paperwork and incident reports as soon as possible while their memories are still fresh. All involved will probably have to give a statement and, in many companies, may have to submit to a drug and alcohol screening. These screenings, even if being done as required by policy, should be done hidden from public view.

Most services have some procedure to review crashes in which their vehicles are involved. The intent of this review is to develop methodologies to identify patterns of dangerous behavior or procedures and provide the ability to share any information from lessons learned to prevent a recurrence. When this information is used to create updated protocols and policies, it may be helpful to ask the following questions:

1. Was a policy of the service violated?
2. Was the vehicle operator at fault?
3. Were there any mitigating factors (e.g., vehicle problem, equipment failure, road hazards)?
4. Has this situation occurred before? If so, what was done in the past?

# Learn from Past Crashes

Agencies can reduce vehicle crashes by researching and learning from past ambulance crashes. Several organizations publish crash investigation reports, including the following:

- National Institute for Occupational Safety and Health (NIOSH), www.cdc.gov/niosh
- National Highway Traffic Safety Administration (NHTSA) Fatality Analysis Reporting System (FARS), www-fars.nhtsa.dot.gov
- EMS Network, www.ems-network.com
- National Transportation Safety Board (NTSB), www.ntsb.gov
- International Association of Fire Chiefs, Firefighter Near Miss, www.firefighternearmiss.com
- EMS Voluntary Event Notification Tool (E.V.E.N.T), event.clirems.org

# Near-Miss Reporting

A near miss is an unplanned event that did not result in injury or damage to an EMS practitioner, vehicle, aircraft, equipment, or patient, but had the potential to do so. Agencies may find it helpful to implement a **near-miss program**, which allows the organization to be aware of close calls that might otherwise go unrecognized. This program can help agencies learn about the circumstances in which near misses occur, which can allow for updates to policies, training, and/or evaluation to address potential issues *before* they can cause real harm.

As with the crash investigation reports, reviewing information on near misses from other jurisdictions is a good way to learn how to prevent the same incidents from happening in your agency. Unlike the NIOSH program for firefighter fatality reporting, no complete national incident reporting system exists for ambulance crashes, injuries, and deaths. The EMS Voluntary Event Notification Tool (E.V.E.N.T.), provided by the Center for Leadership, Innovation, and Research in EMS (CLIR) in partnership with NAEMT, NASEMSO, and the National EMS Management Association, is a voluntary EMS reporting system that EMS personnel are encouraged to use to report incidents. It is designed to improve the safety, quality, and consistent delivery of EMS by collecting and aggregating data submitted anonymously by EMS personnel about near misses involving both patients and practitioners. The subsequent reports can be used to help develop policies, procedures and training programs to improve the safe delivery of EMS. Always follow your department's SOP for reporting incidents and crashes. A model SOP on near-miss reporting has been provided in Chapter 12.

Another source of information on near misses is the International Association of Fire Chiefs (IAFC) National Firefighter Near Miss Reporting System. The database, which has about 10,000 incidents, can be searched for examples of near-miss incidents that can be used in training. While the focus is on near misses in the fire service, reports involving EMS are also included; searching for "ambulance" will bring up reports specific to emergency vehicle operation and safety.

**SAFETY TIP**

**Near-miss recovery** is the effectiveness with which the EVO recovers control of the ambulance after a near miss. In making a split-second response to avoid a crash, it is critical that the EVO is fully familiar with the handling qualities of the ambulance, including its capabilities and limitations. In addition, it is easier to regain control after a near miss if the speed is not excessive and the EVO has been driving to allow for weather, traffic, and roadway conditions.

Although a near miss implies that a crash has been avoided, it does not mean that the danger has completely passed—in recovering from a close call, the EVO must not create another crash risk. Collision avoidance training must stress not simply avoiding a crash, but also ensuring that the actions to avoid the initial crash do not lead to an actual collision.

# SUMMARY

- Defensive driving practices and a safe driving attitude are the keys to avoiding a collision.
- Heinrich's 300-29-1 theory shows just how important it is for an agency to implement training and mitigation of unsafe behavior. Reduce the unsafe behavior and you will reduce the number of collisions before they occur.
- To ensure safety, avoid multitasking or driving too fast for road or weather conditions.
- If the vehicle skids, you should respond by releasing the brakes, allowing the tires to turn, and directing the front wheels in the direction of the skid.
- If the vehicle runs off the roadway, respond slowly to avoid a dangerous overcorrection.
- If a tire fails, slow to a stop and work your way to a safe place on the side of the road.

- It is important to determine the best vehicle position possible at an emergency scene to avoid hazards and ensure that all responders can function appropriately.
- A variety of agencies publish valuable reports on emergency vehicle crashes.
- Emergency vehicle design and safety technology can be used to reduce the likelihood of a collision.
- It is important to know state, local, and agency regulations for how to respond in the event of a collision.
- A near-miss program affords agencies the opportunity to learn from their mistakes.
- Both the CLIR and IAFC have set up near-miss reporting systems that your agency should encourage employees/members to participate in.

# GLOSSARY

**conspicuity** The quality of being clearly discernable and easy to see.

**chevron** An inverted V-shaped striping that slants downward at a 45-degree angle and reflects light; it is applied to the rear of emergency vehicles to increase visibility.

**near-miss program** A system that identifies situations that could have resulted in a collision in an effort to identify necessary revisions in procedures.

**near-miss recovery** The effectiveness with which the EVO recovers control of the ambulance after a near miss.

# ADDITIONAL RESOURCES

Emergency Responder Safety Institute, www.respondersafety.com

EMS Network, www.ems-network.com

Firefighter Near Miss, www.firefighternearmiss.com

*Manual on Uniform Traffic Control Devices (MUTCD)*, mutcd.fhwa.dot.gov

National Highway Traffic Safety Administration (NHTSA) Fatality Analysis Reporting System (FARS), www-fars.nhtsa.dot.gov

National Institute for Occupational Safety and Health (NIOSH), www.cdc.gov/niosh

National Transportation Safety Board (NTSB), www.ntsb.gov

Safety Culture, safetyculture.com

# REFERENCES

Cumberland Valley Volunteer Firemen's Association Emergency Responder Safety Institute. *Study of Protecting Emergency Responders on the Highways and Operation of Emergency Vehicles: A Review of First Responder Agencies Who Have Adopted Emergency Lighting and Vehicle Conspicuity Technology.* June 2018. https://www.respondersafety.com/Download.aspx?id=fa2f464f-2498-4741-917b-809592fcd789

Department of Homeland Security, Science and Technology Directorate. (2013). *First Responders Group, Ambulance Driver Best Practices*, Contract GS-10-F-0181J. Retrieved from https://www.dhs.gov/sites/default/files/publications/Ambulance%20Driver%20%28Operator%29%20Best%20Practices%20Report.pdf

Indiana University Transportation Research Center. (2021, May). *Special Crash Investigations: On-site Ambulance Crash Investigation; Vehicle: 2016 Ford F-350 Type I Ambulance; Location; Oklahoma; Crash Date: August 2017* (Report No. DOT HS 812 943). NHTSA. Retrieved from https://crashstats.nhtsa.dot.gov/Api/Public/ViewPublication/812943

Molnar, J. P. (2010). How to stay safe and avoid crashes. *Journal of Emergency Medical Services*. Retrieved from https://www.jems.com/operations/ambulances-vehicle-ops/how-stay-safe-avoid-crashes/

National Highway Traffic Safety Administration, Office of Emergency Medical Services. (2014). *The National Highway Traffic Safety Administration and ground ambulance crashes.* Retrieved from https://www.naemt.org/Files/HealthSafety/2014%20NHTSA%20Ground%20Amublance%20Crash%20Data.pdf

National Registry of Emergency Medical Technicians. (n.d.). *Resources for EMS professionals.* Retrieved from https://www.nremt.org/Document/resources

Occupational Safety and Health Administration. (2015). *Incident [accident] Investigation: A Guide for Employers, a Systems Approach to Help Prevent Injuries and Illnesses.* Retrieved from https://www.osha.gov/sites/default/files/IncInvGuide4Empl_Dec2015.pdf

Page, D. (2011). Studies show dangers of working in EMS. *Journal of Emergency Medical Services.* Retrieved from https://www.jems.com/operations/studies-show-dangers-working-ems/

Reichard, A., Marsh, S., & Moore, P. (2011). Fatal and nonfatal injuries among emergency medical technicians & paramedics. *Prehospital Emergency Care, 15*(4), 511–517.

U.S. Fire Administration, Federal Emergency Management Agency. (2009). *Emergency vehicle visibility and conspicuity study.* FEMA FA-323. Retrieved from https://www.usfa.fema.gov/downloads/pdf/publications/fa_323.pdf

# CHAPTER 9

# Driving Skills Course

## OBJECTIVES

**9.1** Describe and demonstrate the key components of an emergency vehicle operator (EVO) skills course, including:
  **a.** Physical requirements of the practice space
  **b.** Safety on the skills course
  **c.** Types of skill maneuvers

**9.2** Describe and demonstrate the concepts of:
  **a.** Pretrip inspection
  **b.** Proper seat position for maximum control
  **c.** Proper hand placement on the steering wheel
  **d.** Key components in setting mirrors
  **e.** Proper mirror use
  **f.** Front-end depth perception
  **g.** Rear-end depth perception
  **h.** Left- and right-side judgment
  **i.** Off-tracking and turning

## SCENARIO

You turn on the evening news and hear the following story: A 79-year-old woman in St. Paul, Minnesota, died after she was struck by a fire department ambulance that was backing down an alleyway to reach a patient. The victim was treated by paramedics and was pronounced dead at the scene. The mayor of St. Paul issued a written statement saying that words failed to express city officials' sadness for the woman's family and concern for the anguish of the paramedic crew. The city was undertaking an investigation to determine what happened and what changes need to be implemented to prevent this type of tragedy in the future.

1. What options, other than backing, are generally available when negotiating alleyways?
2. If this incident happened at your department, would standard operating procedures (SOPs) have been violated?
3. If you were involved in a situation such as this, how might it impact your personal reputation, as well as the department's reputation?

## INTRODUCTION

During training, it is important that all EVOs understand how a driving skills course is designed and the reasons behind this design. The driving skills course is an essential component of any successful vehicle operator training program. It is designed to help you understand the dynamics of the vehicle and its relationship to stationary objects around it. During skills training sessions, you will have a chance to perform maneuvers and make mistakes in a supervised setting. The skills course you will be using should ensure that the theoretical and didactic portions of the course are translated into competent and coordinated movement of the vehicle. You can study music and know everything about it, but until you actually pick up an instrument, you will never learn to play. The same can be said for driving an emergency vehicle: You must get behind the wheel and gain hands-on experience. This chapter outlines the basic components that should be included in a driving skills course for EVOs.

## Setting for a Skills Course

The driving sessions should take place in an open area that is large enough to accommodate you and other students working and observing around the course but is blocked off and protected from outside traffic. As you participate in a skills course, you will note that the area needed to perform a single maneuver is at least 10 times the vehicle's length and more than twice its turning radius in width as shown in **Figure 9-1**. In fact, your skills course may be even larger, depending on which maneuvers you will be practicing on the range. Students should use the same vehicles they normally operate when possible. If your agency uses multiple types of vehicles, drivers should be qualified on each one they may operate. The course selected should have safety zones for observations, and there should be no permanent obstacles (e.g., utility poles) on the driving course. Training sessions in the streets may be difficult at first and can lead to a series of problems, especially if the instructor has no control of the vehicle to override any dangerous mistakes. Courses may be physically arranged with stations to work on individual skills or as circuits in which several different types of maneuvers are connected in a series.

### SAFETY TIP

Observers near the driving course should wear high-visibility vests and remain in a designated observation zone to ensure their safety.

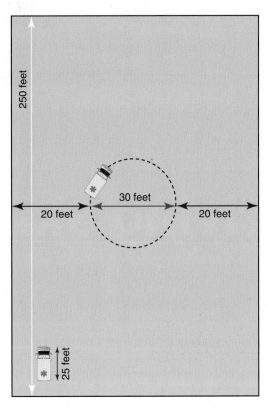

**Figure 9-1** Practice space should have enough room for safe practice of maneuvers, including room to make mistakes and corrections.
© Jones & Bartlett Learning

If the course is used for evening sessions, the location should have proper lighting. Darkness can cause shadows and change the driver's perspective of distance, so it is important to use light towers that are high enough to reduce shadows and bright enough to illuminate the field. Streetlamps or headlights do not provide sufficient lighting and may cast elongated shadows or blinding areas. Though not always possible, training at night can be very valuable to EVOs, but proper lighting is required for everyone's safety. Recommendations for developing SOPs about safety on the driving range are discussed in Chapter 12.

## Before Each Training Session

When beginning a training session, you should start by getting the vehicle ready by inspecting the vehicle and ensuring that the seat and mirrors are positioned properly.

### Vehicle Inspection

The importance of vehicle inspection and maintenance for line units also applies to training units. Just as you will inspect your vehicle at the beginning of a work shift, you should plan to inspect the vehicle before starting any training sessions.

## Seat Positioning

You will need to ensure that the seat is positioned properly before beginning the training session. The seat back should be positioned so you are sitting at a slightly reclined angle, 2 or 3 degrees less than 90 degrees; some students may find this position awkward, but it ensures maximum visibility and control. The seat is contoured so the body fits *into* it and not just against it, which helps to stabilize the driver during sudden changes in direction and acceleration. When the seat back is reclined too much, there is a gap between the seat back and the seat belt, which can lead to excessive body movement, loss of control of the vehicle, and increased risk of injury.

The seat should be positioned so that you can reach both the accelerator and the brake pedal with your legs directly out in front, with a slight bend at the knee. The heel of the right foot should rest on the floor, able to depress both pedals without being lifted. Your chest should be a minimum of 10 inches from the steering wheel, allowing for airbag deployment, and your arms should be close enough to the wheel to have a slight bend in the elbow when holding the wheel at the 9 o'clock and 3 o'clock positions. In this relaxed position, you can use all your upper body muscles if you need to turn the wheel rapidly. Sitting too close to the steering wheel diminishes your range of motion and does not allow for total control of the vehicle. Additionally, if a collision were to occur, the relaxed position can help prevent serious extremity injury, which is more likely to occur when the arms are "locked" and straight.

**SAFETY TIP**

Proper placement of the hands at the 9 o'clock and 3 o'clock positions ensures better handling and stable control of the vehicle when the driver uses shuffle steering, in which the hands are never taken off of the wheel, and helps to reduce the risk of injury following front airbag deployment in the event of a collision.

## Mirror Positioning

Mirrors must be positioned properly to help you know your position relative to your surroundings. When adjusted properly, mirrors will provide a clear view of the road and help you avoid collisions (**Figure 9-2**).

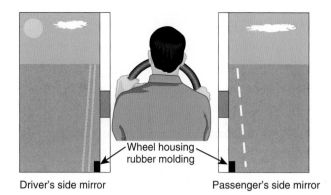

Driver's side mirror                    Passenger's side mirror

**Figure 9-2** Properly adjusted mirrors will ensure a clear view of the road.
© Jones & Bartlett Learning

**SAFETY TIP**

Always take the time to adjust the mirrors when multiple drivers are sharing the same ambulance on the skills course. It may take a minute or two, but it could easily prevent a tragedy on the course.

To correctly adjust the mirrors, you must first be sitting in the proper position. After the seat has been adjusted, sit with good posture to position the mirrors. Adjust the driver's side-view mirror so that the bottom two-thirds of the mirror are below the horizon, with a small sliver of the vehicle on the inside of the mirror and the top of the rear wheel housing in the bottom right (inside) corner. To adjust the passenger's side-view mirror, you should be able to see the top section of the rear wheel housing in the bottom left (inside) corner. In most cases, the passenger's side mirror is convex, which means objects in the mirror are actually closer than they appear.

Mirrors allow the driver to track the vehicle and keep it within the lane on a roadway. They also provide a line of sight to the sides for other obstacles that may block your movements. When driving in the skills course, you should be sure to use your mirrors in a continuous fashion. Scanning your mirrors every 10 seconds allows you to know what is to the sides of you so you can make safe, quick decisions. When turning, you should use both mirrors to ensure you have sufficient clearance. For example, when making a left-hand turn, you should use your left mirror to ensure that you do not sideswipe a vehicle or the center median, and you should use your right mirror to ensure that you do not impact a vehicle that may be trying to go around you.

## Driving with Perspective

One of the most important aspects of the training course is its ability to help the vehicle operator become comfortable with the vehicle. Comfort with the vehicle requires

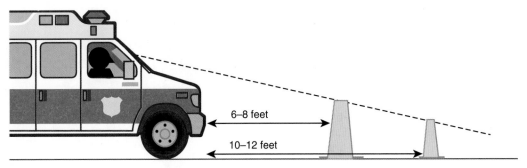

**Figure 9-3** Look past the hood of your vehicle to get a clear view of the big picture.
© Jones & Bartlett Learning

knowing where the vehicle is in relation to other objects and roadway markers; thus, the training course aims to develop the driver's perception of spatial relations.

To help develop a sense of front depth perception, you must first learn the distance between an object and the front of the vehicle. To do so, you should sit in the driver's seat and have an instructor or colleague drag a large cone (approximately 26 to 30 inches tall) toward the vehicle. When you can barely see the top of it, ask the person to stop. Repeat the exercise using a smaller cone (approximately 18 inches tall). Get out and look at the position of the cones in relation to the front of the vehicle. On average, the larger cone will be approximately 6 to 8 feet from the vehicle, and the smaller cone will be 10 to 12 feet from the vehicle (**Figure 9-3**).

Similar judgment is used when backing to determine how far the vehicle can go without striking an object. This time, place a cone beside the rear of the vehicle and another at the farthest point at the rear of the vehicle (usually the step that can't be seen in the rearview mirror) (**Figure 9-4**). You will need to know the full length of the vehicle, not just the box but also the extension of the rear step. If the vehicle has a backup camera, use the large and small cones to show the camera view in relation to the ambulance. This cone exercise will help you understand this spatial relationship between the two cones. With practice, you will be able to back the vehicle safely without striking any objects behind you. It is important to note that all backing in the "real world" should involve a spotter, but that during training on the cone course, backing may be performed without a spotter to help the EVO understand the size of the vehicle and proper maneuvering without worrying about damaging the vehicle or property. Training in spotting (with an instructor acting as the driver) is also helpful so that students can learn how to correctly use hand signals and safely guide the ambulance into position.

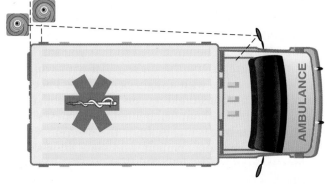

**Figure 9-4** Through understanding the spatial relationship between the two cones, you will be able to avoid backing into an object.
© Jones & Bartlett Learning

Side perception is also important because you will be required to maintain your vehicle in a restricted space, such as a lane of traffic, and position it in narrow spaces. The skills course can help you develop this ability through diminishing lane clearance and tight cornering drills. Drivers need to be aware of how far mirrors and steps stick out from the ambulance.

Turning the vehicle properly will require skills that address **off-tracking**. When a vehicle is traveling straight, the rear wheels should be aligned with (tracking) the front wheels. Off-tracking is what happens to the vehicle when the rear wheels are offset from the front wheels (**Figure 9-5**). Off-tracking can result from issues with the vehicle (e.g., a bent frame or poor wheel alignment), but it also happens routinely when the vehicle is turning. Failure to understand the amount of your vehicle's off-tracking could result in a sideswipe collision, so the skills course should include cornering and handling maneuvers to help you develop a sense of how off-tracking affects your vehicle.

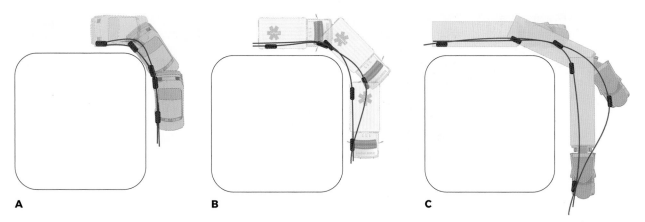

**A**    **B**    **C**

**Figure 9-5** All vehicles have off-tracking. The longer the wheelbase, the wider the track, and the greater the angle that the front wheel can turn all play a part in off-tracking. The colored lines in each diagram demonstrate off-tracking—the purple line indicates the rear wheels, and the green line indicates the front wheels. Notice how the rear wheels take a shorter path than the front wheels of each vehicle: **A.** Sedan. **B.** Type 3 ambulance. **C.** Conventional tractor trailer.
© Jones & Bartlett Learning

The following factors affect the turning angle of a vehicle:

- **Wheelbase** is the measure of the distance from the rear wheel hub to the front wheel hub. The longer the wheelbase, the wider the track and the more of an angle the front wheel can turn.
- **Turning radius** indicates the width of the circle required for the vehicle to turn around without backing up. Take a circle and draw a line to its center: That is the radius. The tighter the turning radius, the wider the off-tracking will be.
- **Vehicle length** is the total length of the vehicle from bumper to bumper.
- **Wheel track** is the measure of the distance from the middle of the tread of the front tire to the middle of the tread of the other front tire; the sharper the angle the wheel can turn, the tighter the turning radius and the wider the off-tracking.

## Skill Maneuvers

Once you have developed a sense of your vehicle and its relationship to your surroundings, you are ready to begin some skill maneuvers to develop vehicle control.

Your instructor should guide you through common skill drills to help you practice skills such as coordinating and timing steering movements, maintaining proper hand position, judging the relationship of fixed objects to the vehicle, using mirrors appropriately, braking smoothly, and improving reaction time (**Table 9-1**).

These drills will give you practice developing vehicle directional control, including the ability to correct for off-tracking and negotiate the vehicle through narrow spaces.

For each maneuver, you may be asked to:

- Enter the maneuver at the required speed
- Keep the vehicle centered
- Check the mirrors
- Place the vehicle in reverse
- Carefully back out of the maneuver
- Control vehicle speed with the brake without bringing the vehicle to a stop until exiting the maneuver

You should receive instructions and a demonstration for each maneuver. To help build your competency and confidence, backing maneuvers on the skills course are performed without a spotter; this is the only time when backing without a spotter is acceptable. A driver should never operate an emergency vehicle without a spotter in real-world conditions.

One example of a maneuver is the switchback. The **switchback maneuver** is a series of sweeping left and right turns that allow the student to develop left- and right-side judgment and front-end depth perception. The maneuver also teaches proper placement into the turn to allow for the off-tracking of the rear wheels without hitting cones with the front end, and it teaches matching of vehicle speed with steering wheel speed (**Figure 9-6**). It is usually completed without brakes. Naturally, the faster you go, the harder it is to perform the maneuver, but it is important to remember this is not a race for completion. Safe, controllable speeds should be maintained at all times.

Your instructor will usually ask you to increase speed over several runs to (1) increase confidence and competency and (2) demonstrate that eventually there is a speed at which it becomes hard to control the ambulance. For example, imagine driving through a parking lot and turning the wheel all the way to the right and

## Table 9-1 Common Skill Drills

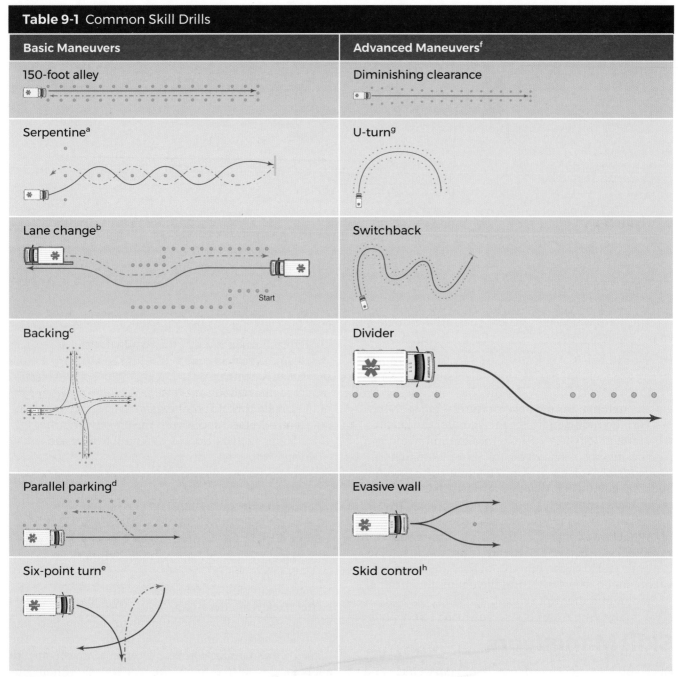

| Basic Maneuvers | Advanced Maneuvers[f] |
|---|---|
| 150-foot alley | Diminishing clearance |
| Serpentine[a] | U-turn[g] |
| Lane change[b] | Switchback |
| Backing[c] | Divider |
| Parallel parking[d] | Evasive wall |
| Six-point turn[e] | Skid control[h] |

→ Forward

← Reverse

[a] < 15 mph with cones 40 feet apart

[b] 15 mph at the decision point

[c] Left, right, and straight

[d] Left and right side

[e] May need spotter

[f] Performing advanced maneuvers may require a larger skills course, additional cones, greater vehicle speeds, and supervision by a more experienced instructor

[g] Left and right

[h] If skid pad is available

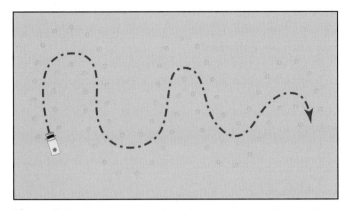

**Figure 9-6** Be sure to allow for safety zones, mistakes, and corrections when performing the switchback maneuver. Turns in the maneuver need to be widened to accommodate vehicle off-tracking and front-end swing.

© Jones & Bartlett Learning

going through a turn; then, when partially through it, you must turn the wheel all the way to the left. The faster you are moving, the more skill will be required.

# Safety Zones

On the training grounds, two different zones should be present. The **maneuvering safety zone** is the area in which the EVO is practicing; these zones should be free of people and any obstacles and allow the student to safely make mistakes and corrections within the skill maneuver. This is the only location in which backing without the use of a spotter is allowed. The other is a **participant safety zone**, which is a safe location for other students on the field waiting for their turn. This particular safety zone needs to be away from the vehicle's trajectory and intended path, which is usually behind a forward moving vehicle and in front of a backing vehicle.

It is also important to have a **safety officer** to oversee all range operations and to ensure all safety practices are adhered to. The safety officer has the ability to shut down operations at a moment's notice until the unsafe situation is rectified.

Remember, SAFETY IS PARAMOUNT! All students and instructors must be paying attention to all areas of the driving field and should not be engaged in idle conversation.

## Monitoring Weather Conditions

Predictable (and unpredictable) weather conditions can hamper driving conditions on the field. Snowfall can cancel or delay driver training operations. Snow removal can diminish the size of the existing course and create unnecessary obstacles. Heavy rain can cause flooding of the course if sufficient drainage isn't provided. Be sure to monitor weather predictions so that adverse weather conditions can be accommodated in advance; this allows the program to be postponed and students redirected back to their respective assignments with minimal negative impact.

Heat and cold conditions must also be taken into account. Standing on a large tarmac in the middle of summer can cause students and staff to rapidly decompensate from the heat. Cooling stations with drinks that contain electrolytes and misting fans can help to keep the program running. Conversely, cold conditions with a light wind blowing over the field can drop windchill temperatures dramatically. Proper clothing and rotating members in and out of heated vehicles can help to protect them. Temperature/humidity index and windchill index charts should be consulted. Most cities and states have predetermined thresholds that suspend all nonemergency outdoor work.

Thunderstorms can pop up when least expected. Lightning, which is the first thunderstorm hazard to arrive and the last to leave, kills more people each year than tornados or hurricanes. If you hear thunder, you should seek shelter; lightning can strike up to 10 miles away from the storm and it strikes the highest grounded object, which is you when you're on the field.

# SUMMARY

- The driving skills course is an essential component of any successful EVO training program.
- Your instructor should design a skills course that has safety zones to allow for mistakes and corrections without colliding with any obstructions.
- When possible, students should use the vehicle or the same type of vehicle they regularly drive.
- Since multiple operators will be training on the same vehicle, it is important to emphasize vehicle

inspection and proper seat and mirror adjustment prior to driving.

- The EVO should develop a level of comfort and experience with the factors that affect the turning angle of the emergency vehicle (i.e., wheelbase, turning radius, vehicle length, and wheel track).
- All of the basic skills maneuvers should be practiced in a safe manner under close supervision by an experienced skills instructor and with a clear safety zone established during the maneuvers.

# GLOSSARY

**maneuvering safety zone** An area where the vehicle operator can make mistakes and attempts at correcting them without the fear of hitting an obstacle.

**off-tracking** The offsetting of the rear wheels of the vehicle from the front wheels, as when the vehicle is turning.

**participant safety zone(s)** Safe locations within the proving ground that keep waiting participants out of the vehicle's trajectory and maneuvers.

**safety officer** An assigned instructor to oversee all aspects of the range maneuvers and the safety of the instructors and students.

**switchback maneuver** A series of sweeping left and right turns that allows the student to develop left- and right-side judgment and front-end depth perception.

**turning radius** The width of the circle required for a vehicle to turn around without backing up.

**vehicle length** The total bumper-to-bumper length of the vehicle.

**wheelbase** The distance from the rear wheel hub to the front wheel hub.

**wheel track** The distance from the middle of the tread of one front tire to the middle of the tread of the other front tire.

# RESOURCES

Lightning safety, https://www.weather.gov/source/zhu/ZHU _Training_Page/lightning_stuff/lightning2/lightning_safety .html

Heat index chart, https://www.weather.gov/ama/heatindex

# CHAPTER 10

# Technological Aids

## OBJECTIVES

**10.1** Identify various technological aids that may be used in emergency response.

**10.2** Explain how to use a global positioning system in emergency vehicle operations.

**10.3** Outline how traffic preemption systems work to assist in emergency response.

**10.4** Discuss how mobile data terminals can be used to assist in communication efforts.

**10.5** Describe how driver behavior monitoring systems can be used to improve emergency vehicle operation.

**10.6** Identify the benefits and potential hazards involved in using technological aids.

**10.7** Discuss the value of new and future developments in EMS technology.

## SCENARIO

Your ambulance is transporting an unstable 68-year-old female patient to the stroke center. You approach an intersection with a red light. As you enter the intersection, you slow down and begin to make eye contact with the other drivers. A car comes barreling into the intersection from your right. You do everything you can to brake and try to steer away, but the car hits your vehicle's rear right quarter panel. Your vehicle is turned onto its side. Both vehicles come to a stop in the intersection.

Your initial concern is for any possible injuries. Fortunately, everyone in your ambulance was wearing their safety restraints, including shoulder restraints on the patient, so no one was hurt. You inform the dispatcher of the need for police, the fire department, and additional ambulances to transport your stroke patient and to check on the other vehicle's occupants. You follow all the steps in your service's SOP on what to do if involved in a crash. Your ambulance will be out of service until it can be repaired, and the car that struck you had significant damage to its front end. The vehicle's driver did not sustain any injuries.

*(continues)*

## INTRODUCTION

Technological devices can be extremely useful in emergency vehicle operations. The modern technological aids discussed in this chapter are used to help the emergency vehicle operator (EVO) find the best route, preempt traffic lights, communicate with dispatch and other emergency medical services (EMS) practitioners, and monitor driver performance. As technology continues to develop, it will be the responsibility of your agency's management to evaluate new products and decide if they are cost effective and will help reduce the probability of crashes while making response safer for EVOs, patients, practitioners, and the public. It will be your responsibility as the EVO to be trained in and fully understand the operations of all technologies that become incorporated into the operation of the emergency vehicle.

However, technological devices are not perfect solutions. We will discuss the dangers of EVOs becoming distracted by or over-reliant upon these devices. For example, just because your vehicle has an automatic backup alarm does not mean you do not have to be aware of who or what is behind the vehicle when backing up. Indeed, many ambulances today have a camera to the rear of the vehicle, yet a small object or child could be missed if you are not careful and do not always use a spotter.

## Global Positioning Systems

A **global positioning system (GPS)** device can be used to accurately identify an object's location. GPS was originally developed in the 1970s by the U.S. Department of Defense for locating ballistic missile submarines, and the same technology is now used to help locate many different objects, such as cellular phones and commercial and private vehicles. This technology relies upon satellites orbiting the earth in precise locations and ground stations that are used to triangulate the GPS device's location (**Figure 10-1**).

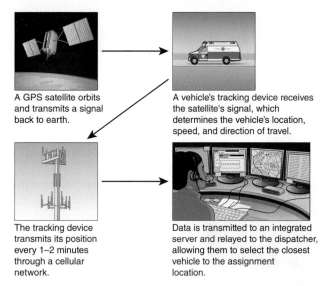

A GPS satellite orbits and transmits a signal back to earth.

A vehicle's tracking device receives the satellite's signal, which determines the vehicle's location, speed, and direction of travel.

The tracking device transmits its position every 1–2 minutes through a cellular network.

Data is transmitted to an integrated server and relayed to the dispatcher, allowing them to select the closest vehicle to the assignment location.

**Figure 10-1** A GPS device enables an EMS agency to track its vehicles and helps crews locate addresses efficiently.
© Jones & Bartlett Learning

In EMS, GPS technology has been combined with global system for mobile communications (GSM) wireless coverage to enable an agency to do the following:

- Track an ambulance's location.
- Allow dispatchers to identify which vehicle is closest to an assignment location to reduce response times.
- Provide quick, efficient directions and rerouting.
- Save money by decreasing fuel costs.
- Use resources more efficiently.

In some agencies without integrated GPS systems, personal navigation devices or smartphone applications may be used (**Figure 10-2**). Typically, the GPS programs on a smartphone involve a very small screen, and they can be a major distraction. Driving while using a cell phone may not even be legal in your state. It is your responsibility as the EVO to understand your state laws. If you have questions, ask police in your jurisdiction.

There are some possible risks to using GPS devices, either integrated or personal, for navigation. First, they may be a distraction to the EVO. Just as you should not be driving and reading the map, the GPS unit can be a distraction, moving your eyes away from the road and mirrors. If possible, your partner should serve as the navigator and guide you based on the GPS or map; this approach will allow you to keep your attention on the road.

In addition, GPS units, computers, and similar devices, depending on their placement in the vehicle, may block a section of the windshield and limit your view. When deciding to use a GPS unit, seriously consider the policies of your service, the size of the GPS screen, and the location of the screen so that it does not interfere with your view of the road, traffic, and mirrors. It should also be easy to hear the directions over the other noises in the cab, such as the siren and communications radios.

> **SAFETY TIP**
>
> Never attempt to program a GPS device while operating the vehicle.

> **SAFETY TIP**
>
> Always follow your agency's standard operating procedures (SOPs) regarding the use of GPS devices.

# Traffic Preemption Systems

**Traffic preemption systems** are a valuable technological aid to EMS response. These systems allow emergency responders to change traffic signals to allow them to clear an intersection and gain right-of-way. They rely on a series of receivers purchased by the municipality and installed at intersections with traffic lights, and emitters that are installed on the emergency vehicle (**Figure 10-3**). When an emergency vehicle is responding to an assignment and approaches an intersection equipped with a

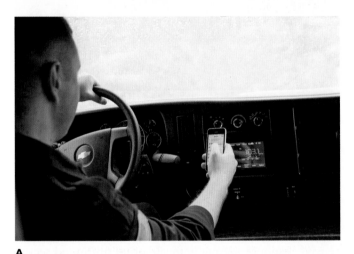

A

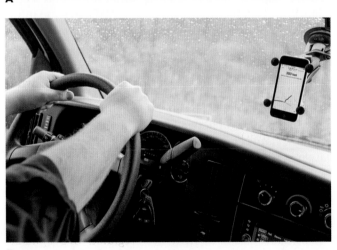

B

**Figure 10-2** Personal GPS devices may be permitted by some agencies to assist with navigation. **(A)** Unmounted they are a distraction, and **(B)** mounted they are less distracting.

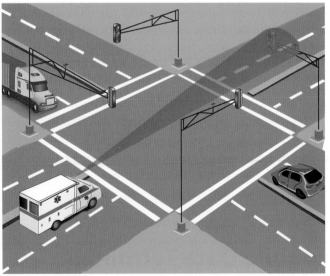

**Figure 10-3** Traffic preemption systems work using infrared beams to trigger traffic lights to change, giving the emergency vehicle the exclusive right-of-way.

traffic preemption system, the traffic light is preempted from its regular pattern. It will cycle through the caution (yellow) and red lights for all other directions, giving the green light and exclusive right-of-way to the emergency vehicle. This helps to clear the path in front of the emergency vehicle, which in turn can reduce response time. These systems can theoretically reduce the likelihood of collisions by giving the emergency vehicle the right-of-way, although their effectiveness depends on the volume of traffic and how long the emergency vehicle will be on the pathway being cleared by a series of green lights instead of the occasional red light.

Preemption priority is set so that if more than one emergency vehicle is approaching the intersection from different directions at the same time, only one will have the green light to proceed. Some systems include a flood light that notifies the public and other emergency vehicles of the direction of the emergency vehicle's approach as well as to confirm that the device has been activated. It is important to note that not all emergency vehicles are equipped with traffic preemption emitters. Therefore, it could happen that even if you have the right-of-way from your traffic preemption device, there could be another nonequipped vehicle attempting to proceed through the same intersection from a different direction. You should always use caution proceeding through the intersection, even with a traffic preemption device installed.

These devices can also be beneficial to patient care when they are used properly. Some services allow them to function independently of the emergency warning devices for transporting patients who are experiencing a time-critical event where a quiet ride is necessary (keeping patients calm, such as in cases of heart attack). Using preemption devices allows the transporting ambulance to move efficiently through traffic but decreases the risk associated and the stress response the patient may have to emergency transport. This technology is not available on all vehicles, so be sure to follow your agency's SOPs and know your vehicle.

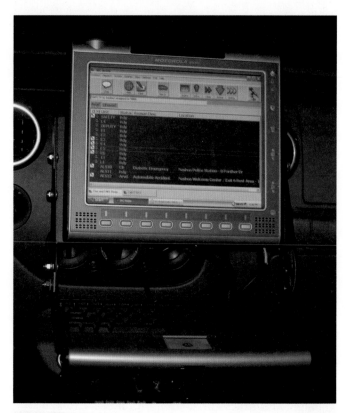

**Figure 10-4** Mobile data terminals are a great resource for communication, planning, and reporting.
Courtesy of the City of Nashua, New Hampshire

> **SAFETY TIP**
>
> Traffic preemption systems are useful, but they do not remove your responsibility to ensure that the intersection is clear.

# Mobile Data Terminals

A **mobile data terminal (MDT)** is an in-vehicle communication device that has become the standard for many EMS agencies and emergency responders (**Figure 10-4**). Most MDTs are a part of the computer-aided dispatch (CAD) system and extend the CAD capabilities. Some services utilize an in-vehicle laptop computer (mobile data computer, or MDC) that is mounted in the cab of the ambulance. These terminals or laptops can provide extensive response mapping, locate other units, and secure real-time access to public databases. MDTs increase information sharing and facilitate delivery of mission-critical information to the field (e.g., location of hazardous materials, building plans, and emergency plans). Many of the newer systems can provide electronic patient care report (e-PCR) capabilities and billing information and can even be used for continuing education while the unit is posted at a location between calls. Some also use buttons to mark status changes to limit radio traffic, especially in larger systems.

MDTs are typically mounted in the cab between the seats, providing easy access to both the passenger and the EVO. Placement of the devices must not interfere with the vehicle's airbag system. MDTs should never be used by the EVO during vehicle operation, as doing so would distract the operator from driving duties. Also, depending on where they are mounted, they may create a blind spot or vision issues at night due to their bright screens. Always follow your agency's SOPs regarding MDT use.

# Driver Behavior Monitoring Systems

In the past, supervisors would have to accompany crews on the road to monitor driver performance or rely on observations and anecdotal evidence from other personnel to determine if EVOs were using safe driving techniques. However, this process of evaluation was inefficient, subjective, and unpredictable. Now, electronic **driver monitoring devices** can be used to monitor driver performance and help prevent collisions. These devices are also referred to as **driver behavior monitoring systems (DBMSs)**. NFPA 1901 requires a video data recording device (or **black box**) on all apparatus purchased after January 1, 2010. Variables such as vehicle speed, acceleration, deceleration, engine throttle position, antilock braking system, whether a seat is occupied, and if the occupant is seat-belted will be monitored. Software to produce reports on these behaviors is also required.

Driver monitoring devices record the driver's behavior, provide immediate feedback to the driver, and analyze the data to let the organization know the driver's overall compliance to driving standards. They are valuable resources for evaluating and addressing any problems in driver performance. Using these monitoring devices, management may be able to determine which drivers need additional guidance and training before problems occur. In many cases, electronic monitoring can be used as evidence of a driver's innocence in the event of a collision.

Several different types of monitoring systems are available for EMS vehicles as shown in **Figure 10-5**. While there are some differences in how the specific devices work, the general concept is the same. They use data recording devices such as video cameras and/ or sensors to record the vehicle's location, forward and lateral movement, and driver activities (**Figure 10-6**). In the event of any unexpected movement, such as a collision, quick acceleration, or sharp turn, the device will record information about the event, including use of turn signals, vehicle position and speed, and vehicle mechanical states (e.g., brake pressure, RPMs, etc.). The data may be provided as real-time feedback to the driver and/or supervisors or may be analyzed by the manufacturer, with feedback later provided to the agency. The driver may be notified of behavior that is considered unacceptable or that an event has been recorded by a light on the device or an audible tone.

Management can review the recorded data with the EVO to provide further information or training regarding the event. Quality assurance personnel can maintain database files that track and cross-check different types of events, frequency of events, and event details such as certain time of day and weather conditions. Your

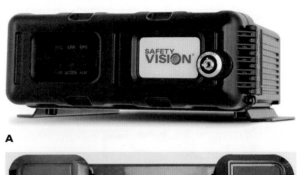

**A**

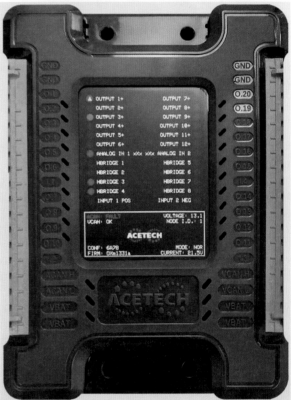

**B**

**Figure 10-5** Sample driver behavior monitoring systems. **A.** Safety Vision. **B.** ACETECH.

**A:** © Safety Vision, LLC; **B:** Courtesy of ACETECH.

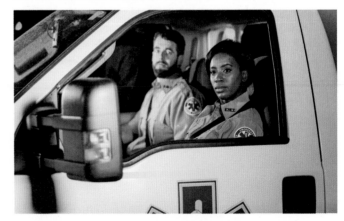

**Figure 10-6** Monitoring devices can record drivers' actions. The EVO may hear an audible tone if driving too quickly.

© kali9/E+/Getty Images

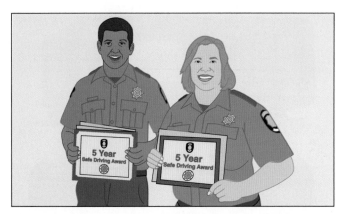

**Figure 10-7** Rewarding personnel is one way to reinforce good driving habits.
© Jones & Bartlett Learning

service's driving instructor may share with members/employees in their emergency vehicle operator course some clips taken from these recording devices, noting specific lessons to learn from.

It is important to note that data from monitoring devices can serve as evidence to support the emergency vehicle operator in the event of a collision, and that the devices may also be used to provide safe drivers with positive feedback. Management can recognize personnel who are not involved in events that trigger the system and reward them for their safe driving habits (**Figure 10-7**).

These devices may be cost prohibitive for some services. However, research has shown that use of driver monitoring systems can improve EVO performance, with associated cost savings from the reduced need for maintenance and driver retraining. Also, because the evidence can show that companies were operating safely, legal costs associated with liability issues may be decreased. Some insurance companies may offer discounts for vehicles that use these devices, another way in which a driver monitoring system can pay for itself over time.

# The Next Generation of EMS Technology

Since the new products in development are usually significant investments by the developing manufacturers, there is little information on what devices are currently in development. One can only speculate that the systems in the ambulance will give us more computer-monitored feedback on the condition of the vehicle, its lights and compartments, and its handling, not to mention the changes in how we access and transmit patient information. Just look at the advances in automobiles. Beyond the demands of customers, federal and nonprofit agencies have developed guidelines to increase safety, which influence design decisions. There are guidance systems available in cars today that warn drivers when they are approaching danger and begin to slow their vehicle before a crash occurs. More sophisticated GPS systems can alert drivers to traffic backups and advise alternate routes. There are even systems that will parallel park an automobile. In the large trucks, adaptive cruise control will maintain a safe following distance behind the vehicle in front of the truck, and collision mitigation systems will slow the vehicle when there is danger of a collision. Artificial intelligence (AI) is also quickly emerging as a new technology in many fields. At this point, it is still unknown the effect AI could have on emergency services and the EVO. Stay tuned!

However, increased use of technology has not necessarily resulted in a reduction in collisions. The reason for this is that you cannot completely correct driver behavior with technological solutions. The prevalence of touch screens means less tactile feedback to the user, which results in drivers needing to look at the devices (and take their eyes off of the road) to operate them. Safety features, such as backup cameras and blind-spot indicators, can lead to driver complacency and the assumption that if the system does not alert to a hazard, then a hazard must not exist. Overreliance on GPS has shown to negatively impact spatial awareness and ability to self-navigate.

Technology, while helpful, can only work in conjunction with an alert, trained operator who uses these devices as *part* of their overall approach to safety, not their *entire* approach. Technology can also fail without warning, or access can be limited due to disasters or the overloading of communications systems, so EVOs need to know how to navigate their response area and safely operate their vehicles without technological assistance. Advances in medical technology have allowed EMS practitioners to provide more care in the field, but new equipment is useless without the foundational knowledge and skills of assessment and treatment. Like automated external defibrillators, GPS and traffic exemption devices are simply tools to help you do your job, but you still need to know how to use them. Technology is only useful when it is used correctly.

# SUMMARY

- Technology can be useful and improve response and safety, but it also has its limitations. Improvements such as backup cameras cannot replace an actual spotter.
- Global positioning system (GPS) units, mobile data terminals/computers (MDTs/MDCs), and other mapping devices have made responding easier, but they also can be distractions for the driver.
- As much as possible, the passenger should be responsible for navigation and communicating with dispatch so the EVO can focus on the task of driving.
- Traffic preemption systems work to assist in emergency response by giving emergency vehicles the right-of-way at intersections.

- MDTs or MDCs can provide valuable run information on the location of and hazards involved in a call and can even track ambulances' status without use of the radio.
- Driver monitoring systems can give feedback to drivers and agencies that can be used to correct risky and dangerous behaviors as well as reward safe driving habits.
- Each new type of technology should be evaluated for both its potential benefits and its limitations.

# GLOSSARY

**black box** A monitoring recorder, found on commercial aircraft, also called a flight recorder. Similar types of electronic devices are often found in emergency vehicles to provide a recording of events leading up to the moments when a crash occurred.

**driver behavior monitoring systems (DBMSs)** See *driver monitoring devices.*

**driver monitoring devices** Monitoring systems that track driver actions, vehicle movement, and immediate

environment around the vehicle using video cameras and sensors.

**global positioning system (GPS)** Satellite-based location and navigation system used to locate vehicles and provide directions to specific locations.

**mobile data terminal (MDT)** A computerized device similar to a laptop computer that is used to communicate with a central dispatch office.

**traffic preemption systems** Systems used to preempt traffic lights, giving emergency vehicles the right-of-way.

# REFERENCES

Dahmani, L., & Bohbot, V. D. (2020). Habitual use of GPS negatively impacts spatial memory during self-guided navigation. *Science Reports, 10*(1), 6310.

Department of Homeland Security, Science and Technology Directorate, First Responders Group. (2013). *A research study of ambulance operations and best practice considerations for emergency medical services personnel.* Retrieved from https://www.dhs.gov/sites/default/files/publications/Ambulance%20Driver%20%28Operator%29%20Best%20Practices%20Report.pdf

Levick, N. R., & Swanson, J. An optimal solution for enhancing ambulance safety: implementing a driver performance feedback and monitoring device in ground emergency medical service vehicles. Presented at the 49th Annual Proceedings Association for the Advancement of Automotive Medicine, September 12–14, 2005.

U.S. Department of Transportation, ITS Joint Program Office (2006). *Traffic signal preemption for emergency vehicles: a cross-cutting study.* FHWA-JPO-05-010. Retrieved from https://rosap.ntl.bts.gov/view/dot/3655/dot_3655_DS1.pdf

# CHAPTER 11

# Simulation Training

## OBJECTIVES

**11.1** Describe the value of simulation training in emergency vehicle operations.

**11.2** Explain how a driving simulator can be used in emergency vehicle operator (EVO) training.

**11.3** Discuss how virtual reality is used in simulator training.

## SCENARIO

Miguel had just graduated from his emergency medical technician (EMT) program. After several weeks of training, he was finally allowed to drive the ambulance. When a call came in for a cardiac patient in critical condition, he engaged the lights and siren and proceeded to the call carefully, clearing traffic along the way. As he approached a busy intersection, he tried to remember everything he was supposed to do. He remembered to pull left of center and proceed up to the intersection against the red light. He remembered to ease his way into the intersection, recognizing that the two lanes of traffic to his left had yielded the right-of-way. Miguel proceeded to the double yellow line and saw that the truck in the lane immediately to his right had stopped to yield the right-of-way as well.

Before his training, Miguel would have felt confident that this situation was safe and would have proceeded through the intersection, but during his simulation training, Miguel had encountered a very similar situation that caused him to now pause for a moment. The truck beside him was large and in a position to block his view of the second lane of traffic. He knew from simulation that there could be another vehicle approaching from the right that he could not see. So, he moved forward slowly, allowing his lights and siren to warn oncoming traffic and waited to be sure the intersection was truly clear before proceeding. When he pulled

*(continues)*

through the intersection, he saw the truck indeed had been concealing a smaller vehicle that had stopped, but easily could have collided with the ambulance if it had not heard the siren. In a simulation he could make a mistake, analyze the action, and change his behaviors so he would not make that potentially fatal mistake when out on the street. Miguel was grateful his simulation training had prepared him for this situation, and he proceeded safely through the intersection to the call.

1. Do you use simulation in driving training?
2. Typically, your first attempt at airway management and other such skills will be performed on simulators. Should the approach to driving skills be the same? Explain your reasoning.
3. Are there other aspects of emergency medical services (EMS) that are as risky as emergency driving?

## INTRODUCTION

Emergency vehicle operation requires a foundation of solid basic driving skills and a clear understanding of vehicle and traffic dynamics. To achieve this goal, many EMS services are using simulators to provide an interactive learning environment where students can role-play in a realistic situation and learn from their mistakes. Simulation training allows EVOs to synthesize the knowledge they have learned in their lectures, the motor skills they have developed in training, and the judgment they have acquired in their skills courses (**Figure 11-1**).

With the help of technology, EMS agencies can now use simulation modules to replicate a series of complex events, just as the military, airline industry, and medical field have for their specialized training. Simulation allows students to gain "on the job" training in a supervised setting where no one gets hurt and no property is damaged. It is valuable training that helps EVOs minimize collisions and maximize recognition and avoidance of hazards. In New York City, after services implemented driving simulation in their EVO training, intersection collisions decreased significantly. Any reduction in crashes likely more than pays for the cost of the simulation equipment and the training program required.

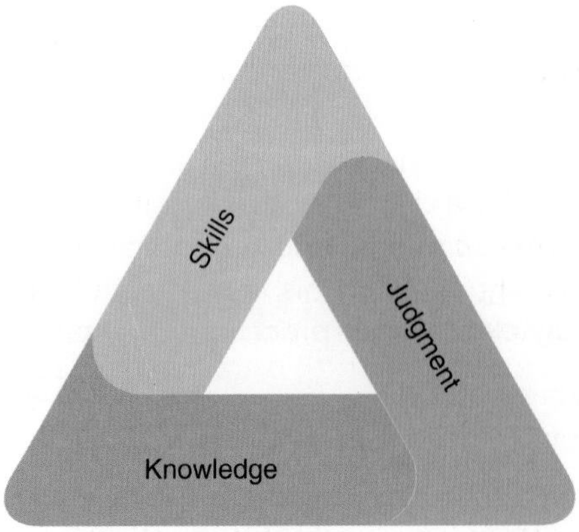

Thanks to gaming systems, today's young adults have been using simulation computer games since they were children. They are very familiar with the hand–eye coordination it takes to play these games and are comfortable and quick learners in a simulated environment. Many of today's EVOs have played driving games in the past. Some of the learning tools on the market today build on that knowledge base. For example, one company has produced a game-like computer exercise with the goal of improving reaction time, reducing crash risk, and increasing control in various driving conditions.

## Driving Simulators

In a simulation training session, you will be practicing a realistic scenario using a **driving simulator**. Driving simulators are used in driver's education courses taught in educational training centers. They can also be used for research purposes to assess driver behavior and human factors. They present an opportunity for the student to safely experience road conditions, traffic conditions, and hazards, and some can even recreate actual collisions. Once the student gets behind the wheel of a simulator and receives some simple instructions in operating the "vehicle," the exercise can be challenging and fun at the same time.

Simulators used in EMS training are designed to mimic the department's regular emergency vehicles and should have full functionality (i.e., steering, gas, brakes, turning radius, stopping distance, and center of gravity of an actual EMS vehicle) (**Figure 11-2**). A single simulator can be used to mimic several different types of vehicles. Simulators may be open or enclosed cab units consisting of a driver's seat, dash console, steering wheel, pedals, siren, radio, and so on. The field of vision resembles a true driving environment, reflecting the view a driver would see through the windshield, windows, and mirrors,

**Figure 11-1** The triangle of training.

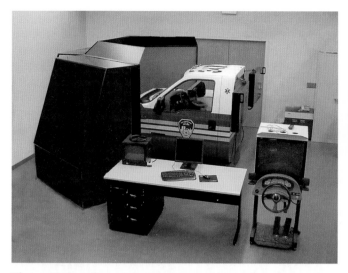

**Figure 11-2** Fully enclosed simulators can mimic many different types of emergency vehicles.
© Jones & Bartlett Learning. Courtesy of FAAC, Inc.

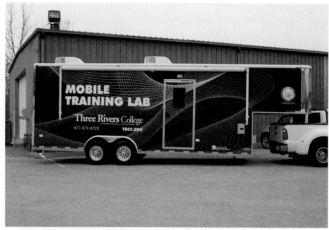

**Figure 11-4** Mobile simulators can be brought to your agency or training location.
Courtesy of Jack Armor and Three Rivers Community College

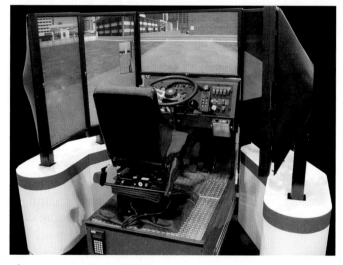

**Figure 11-3** Driving simulators on a motion-based platform can help provide training in vehicle dynamics.
© Jones & Bartlett Learning. Courtesy of FAAC, Inc.

**SAFETY TIP**

Similar to how mannequins allow first-time EMS practitioners to safely practice clinical skills, simulators allow EVOs to gain valuable driving experience without the consequences of real driving.

including blind spots. Driving simulators usually have a motion-based component that enables students to feel the inertia and dynamics of the vehicle (**Figure 11-3**). The more realistic and closer to the handling and feel of the actual emergency vehicles that students will be using on the job, the less likely students will be to rationalize away performance as "only a function of using the simulator"; that is, they will be less likely to feel that their actions would be different if they were on the streets in their community in an actual emergency vehicle.

Your agency may send you to a training center for your simulation training or may arrange for mobile simulators at your site (**Figure 11-4**).

Like video games, simulations use **virtual reality** in which EVOs can practice new skills without repercussions. Virtual reality takes the form of a computer-based simulated environment through which users can interact with one another and their surroundings. Most simulators will provide a variety of virtual worlds to mimic urban areas, congested streets, rural countryside, gravel roads, highways, and so on (**Figure 11-5**). In these virtual worlds, students are given freedom to choose which direction to go, how fast to go, and what to do, and they can practice the skills they have learned, such as intersection analysis or soft shoulder recovery, without putting themselves and other drivers in danger.

Many of these simulators utilize geospecific mapping technologies such as those used in global positioning system (GPS) mapping. The following technologies are fundamental to the creation of virtual environments:

- A **geographic information system (GIS)** is a computer system that combines database management system functionality with location information. A GIS can capture, manage, integrate, manipulate, analyze, and display data that are spatially referenced to the earth's surface.

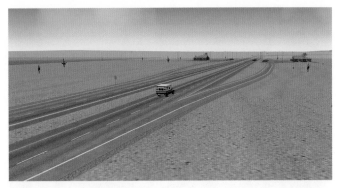

A

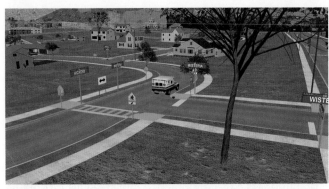

B

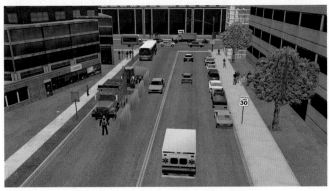

C

**Figure 11-5** Virtual reality can be programmed to mimic **(A)** rural, **(B)** suburban, or **(C)** urban driving environments.

© Jones & Bartlett Learning. Courtesy of FAAC, Inc.

- **Georeferencing** is the process of determining the location of data in physical space. This process often involves converting geographic data to a real-world coordinate system.
- *GPS* is a system based on satellites that allows a user with a receiver to determine precise coordinates for their location on the earth's surface. GPS mapping is a primary source of spatial data—that is, data that define a location.

These technologies can even be used to recreate existing environments, such that students could practice responding in a virtual version of their response area or other real-world location.

Simulators can also mimic various weather situations, such as rain, snow, fog, ice, wind, and bright sun, so you can practice driving in adverse conditions and with limited visibility. They can also present various traffic patterns so you can work on handling your vehicle in relationship to other motor vehicles, pedestrians, and/ or animals running across the road. Your instructor may join in your simulation, controlling various entities such as other motorists and interacting with you to work on specific skills or situations.

## Active Versus Passive Training

Broadly speaking, there are two main ways in which students are taught: passive training and active training. In **passive training**, students are provided with information that they then internalize. **Active training**, in contrast, requires the student to apply the information they have acquired. Students learn in different ways, so using multiple approaches can help with knowledge retention and reinforce key points (**Figure 11-6**). In the case of emergency vehicle training, the EVO would first learn basic concepts, such as the effects of rain on road conditions via a lecture or text, and then would be tested on that knowledge by having to demonstrate how they would respond in a simulated thunderstorm.

As a form of active training, simulation is powerful because it allows for the development of **recognition-primed decision making (RPDM)**. RPDM is a process for how people can quickly make effective decisions in complex situations. It involves applying lessons learned from past experiences to current situations, streamlining the decision-making process by limiting options to those that have worked previously. Simulation can help learners with decision making by presenting a situation, allowing the brain to develop a response that is consistent with the event, and eliminating much of the trial and error of guessing what to do the next time the situation occurs.

Simulation also allows for training for low probability/ high impact events, which are events that occur infrequently but can have devastating consequences (such as terrorist attacks and natural/man-made disasters). By preparing and training for these emergencies, we can take a complex emergency and make it into a set of procedures to follow, like a vehicle inspection checklist or treatment algorithm. This reduces the amount of decision making required on the part of the EVO, which, in turn, reduces the chance of mistakes.

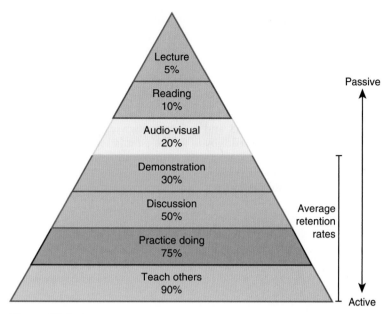

**Figure 11-6** The learning pyramid.

## SUMMARY

- Simulation training in emergency vehicle operations is valuable because it allows the EVO to experience the dangers and challenges of emergency driving without the consequences.

- Driving simulators can be used to teach most emergency maneuvers, mechanical failures, tire blowouts, and other driving issues so that when they happen in the real world, it is not the first time the EVO is experiencing the situation.

- Virtual reality is used in simulation training to create a realistic environment for EVOs so they can react to real-life situations in a simulation.

- Generally, both passive and active training methods are used in EVO education. Active training using simulations is especially useful, as it helps develop recognition-primed decision making for what are normally rare events.

## GLOSSARY

**active training** The portion of training in which a student develops the answers through facilitated learning instead of instruction.

**driving simulator** A training tool used in driver's education courses to expose students to realistic driving situations and to assess driver behavior and human factors. Typically, simulators involve a computer display of everything the operator would see through the windshield and mirrors during actual driving.

**geographic information system (GIS)** A computer system that combines database management system functionality with location information.

**georeferencing** The process of determining the location of data in physical space.

**passive training** The portion of training in which a student receives instruction and is expected to glean knowledge from it rather than develop the knowledge on their own.

**recognition-primed decision making (RPDM)** A process for how people can quickly make effective decisions in complex situations; based on using prior experiences to predict possible outcomes.

**virtual reality** A computer-based simulated environment through which users can interact with one another and their environment.

## REFERENCES

Centers for Disease Control and Prevention. (2019). GIS and public health at CDC. Retrieved from https://www.cdc.gov/gis/index.htm

Raheb, R. (2011, March 22). Driver training simulation: Measuring a return on your investment. *FireRescue1*. Retrieved from https://www.firerescue1.com/fire-products/training-products/fire-simulation/driving-simulation/articles/driver-training-simulation-measuring-a-return-on-your-investment-ZBKk5wWTmAVTjTmF/

# CHAPTER 12

# Standard Operating Procedures

## OBJECTIVES

**12.1** Explain the general process used to develop a standard operating procedure (SOP).

**12.2** Describe key concepts to incorporate in an SOP for backing an EMS vehicle.

**12.3** Discuss key concepts to incorporate in an SOP for the use of safety restraints.

**12.4** Review key points to include in an emergency lighting at the scene SOP.

**12.5** Describe key concepts to incorporate in an SOP for driving range safety.

**12.6** Describe key concepts to incorporate in an SOP on encountering a collision.

**12.7** Describe key concepts to incorporate in an SOP for a crash involving an EMS vehicle.

**12.8** Discuss key concepts to incorporate in an SOP for visibility at the scene of an emergency call.

**12.9** Describe key concepts to incorporate in a sample SOP on qualifications for new EVOs.

**12.10** Describe key concepts to incorporate in an SOP for the avoidance of distractions while driving.

**12.11** Describe key concepts to incorporate in an SOP for alcohol and drug use.

**12.12** Describe key concepts to incorporate in an SOP on reporting work-related injuries/illnesses and near-misses.

## SCENARIO

You and your partner are dispatched to an unconscious patient on the opposite side of town, on a street with which neither of you is familiar. You race out of the station urgently, without checking the map, since your agency recently installed a new global positioning system (GPS) navigation device in your unit. It is late afternoon, the sky is clear, the sun is bright and shining, and the roads are dry. Once in the ambulance, you engage your lights and siren, due to the priority of the call, and start down Main Street. It is a two-way street with cars parallel parked on both sides, so you keep a lookout for pedestrians.

You now need to use the new GPS unit and reach over to turn it on. You have one hand on the wheel as you are entering the address into the GPS unit, when suddenly you look up at the road and notice the ambulance

*(continues)*

## SCENARIO (CONTINUED)

has veered about 2 feet to the right and is approaching a parked flatbed truck. You see it and apply the brakes, but it is too late.

The collision happens with such force that it tears off the right doors and sidewalls of the ambulance. The windshield breaks, shattering glass all over the front cab. Your partner is unconscious, and there is blood all over the inside of the front cab of the Type II ambulance.

You shut off the motor of the ambulance and immediately call the dispatcher to request the police, reassignment of your original call to another unit, and an ambulance for your partner. You exit the vehicle and go over to care for your partner whose right arm appears to be severely torn from the shoulder and is bleeding profusely. You can hear sirens in the background from the approaching ambulance.

1. When new technology is introduced in your department, what type of training should take place?
2. Can a GPS or navigation system replace sound knowledge of your response zone and preplanning a route?
3. Should an EMS agency have an SOP regarding the proper use of the GPS and route preplanning?

## INTRODUCTION

Each state has its own set of motor vehicle laws, and local municipalities and departments often have their own, more specific, regulations as well. In addition to these rules, an emergency medical services (EMS) agency should have its own guidelines, known as **standard operating procedures (SOPs)**. An SOP is a very specific guideline designed to clarify or enhance state and local laws as well as describe the step-by-step procedures that management expects all personnel to follow to safely accomplish a specific job. These policies in many cases will carry the weight of the law.

For example, state law may allow an emergency vehicle operator (EVO) to be exempt from following the posted speed limit when operating an emergency vehicle during an emergency operation. The local law may have a posted speed limit of 30 mph. However, if the state does not limit the speed of an emergency vehicle during a response, then there is no cap on the rate of travel according to the state. Beyond expecting the EVOs to take full responsibility for all of their actions, an agency may wish to create an SOP on this issue. Some agencies have developed SOPs designed to cap or limit the speed of their vehicles (e.g., no more than 20 mph over the posted speed limit). SOPs can be legally binding, and it is your responsibility to be familiar with your agency's SOPs and follow them. (See Chapter 3 for more on the legal considerations of SOPs.)

In this chapter we will discuss how SOPs are developed and their importance to every member of the organization. We will provide some key features of effective SOPs that every agency should seriously consider implementing if they do not already have an SOP on the specific topic.

## SAFETY TIP

EVOs must be compliant with the laws in their state and local jurisdictions as well as all agency SOPs.

# How SOPs Are Developed

Since the EVO will need to follow SOPs in their agency, it is helpful to understand how they are developed. First there needs to be a topic or issue needing direction and/or clarification in which an SOP could be helpful. The officer, committee, or members who are empowered to develop the SOP should clearly define the problem or subject that needs to be addressed. (In our discussion here, we will pretend that you are the person charged with creating the new SOP.) Next, consider why the SOP is being developed and the need for its development. It takes time to develop a new policy, and it should not be an overreaction to an issue involving a single member or employee that could be better dealt with by meeting directly with the individual. Unfortunately, there are many

## SAFETY TIP

When developing a policy, you should first define the **SMART objectives** of the policy. The acronym SMART is used to describe the key characteristics of meaningful objectives: *specific, measurable, achievable, realistic,* and *time*-bound.

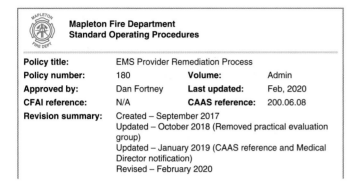

| Policy title: | EMS Provider Remediation Process | | |
|---|---|---|---|
| Policy number: | 180 | **Volume:** | Admin |
| Approved by: | Dan Fortney | **Last updated:** | Feb, 2020 |
| CFAI reference: | N/A | **CAAS reference:** | 200.06.08 |
| Revision summary: | Created – September 2017<br>Updated – October 2018 (Removed practical evaluation group)<br>Updated – January 2019 (CAAS reference and Medical Director notification)<br>Revised – February 2020 | | |

**Figure 12-1** Sample heading for a department/agency SOP.
Courtesy of the City of Rogers, Arkansas

**Table 12-1** Comparison of Skills with Possible SOPs

| Skill | SOP |
|---|---|
| Operation of lights and siren | When use of lights and siren is permitted |
| Vehicle operation during inclement weather | Maximum allowed speeds based on weather conditions |
| How to use communications equipment | Protocols regarding EVOs use of equipment during vehicle operation |
| Steps in navigating an intersection | Role of passenger in clearing an intersection |
| Fatigue avoidance methods | Guidelines to remove an EVO from duty when fatigued |
| How to park the vehicle | Vehicle placement at different scenes |

policies in many organizations that were developed in this manner rather than dealing with the specific person who caused the problem. Remember, once it becomes the policy of your agency, everyone will need to become familiar with the SOP and follow it.

Next do some research on the topic. Usually, a problem identified in your agency has been identified in other agencies, so it is helpful to ask around and see samples of how other organizations chose to resolve the issue. Obtain copies of other agencies' SOPs on the specific topic to see how they dealt with the problem. You are not bound to solve your agency's problems in the same manner as agencies that are different than yours but you certainly can borrow those agencies' best ideas, often referred to as "best practices." After defining the problem and analyzing the other available SOPs, it is time to write a first draft. It will be helpful to circulate the draft (clearly marked as "draft") to a representative group of your members and management to ask them for their feedback on the clarity of the SOP and suggestions for improvements. If your agency has a legal counsel, you should ask for input to make sure the new SOP does not violate any laws and will be enforceable within your organization. Most agencies have a numbering system for their SOPs so they can be easily indexed by subject and located in a SOP manual quickly. The SOP should clearly state who it is issued by and the date it becomes effective, as illustrated in **Figure 12-1**.

It is always helpful to get the input of the members or employees so the final version of the SOP can have ownership, buy-in, and a commitment from them to learn and follow the new SOP. Take the time to issue all members or employees a copy of the SOP and provide training as needed. After an SOP has been implemented, consider a review of all SOPs on a regular (e.g., annual) basis to see if they are still relevant, warranted, and effective.

An SOP is not designed to replace training or technical skills, but rather to provide guidance on when and how to use those skills. **Table 12-1** provides a list of common skills the EVO should possess with examples of related SOP topics.

# Be Familiar with Your Agency's SOPs

EVOs must learn and fully comply with their agencies' SOPs just as they are expected to follow the rules of the road. Some services have a limited number of SOPs, which they train in and have come to believe in as the accepted standard of behavior for their service. Other agencies have volumes of SOPs, which most of their members or employees do not remember. Since all will be held up to the policy should there be a legal action, it is best to have fewer policies that everyone fully understands and complies with. Just as all EMS practitioners have to learn and follow the treatment protocols, all EVOs should be required to learn and follow the service's vehicle operation SOPs. If you must refer to a pocket guide or online version until you commit them to memory, then do it that way. At the very least, bring a copy with you to work and review them until you are familiar with them. Employers need to make sure the most updated SOPs are available to all personnel and that everyone receives updates, and the appropriate training as needed, if they are changed.

# Recommendations for Policies

There is no one list of SOP topics that is suitable for all agencies—SOPs will vary based on service area, population demographics, number of employees and their training level (basic vs. advanced life support practitioners), and mutual/automatic aid response, among other considerations. However, the Federal Emergency Management Agency and the U.S. Fire Administration have come up with a list of general topics for agencies to consider when creating and evaluating their own SOPs, which can be found at the end of this chapter in **Appendix 12-A**. While some of the topic areas may seem more relevant to the fire service, if your agency regularly responds to incidents alongside the fire department, it may be worthwhile to consider creating SOPs to address these situations. For example, if your jurisdiction includes a chemical processing plant or large outdoor recreation area, SOPs related to hazardous materials response or wilderness rescue could prove useful.

The remainder of this chapter provides recommendations to incorporate into the development of specific SOPs on the following topics:

- Backing of the emergency vehicle
- Seat belts and restraints in the emergency vehicle
- Use of emergency lights at an incident on a roadway
- Safety procedures on the driving range
- Postcollision guidelines
- Encountering a collision
- Visibility at the scene
- Qualifications for new EVOs
- Avoidance of distractions while driving
- Alcohol and drug use
- Reporting work-related injuries/illnesses and near misses

Most of these recommendations come from SOPs that have already been developed and are in place in organizations across the United States today. Rather than including specific agencies' SOPs as models, since there are so many excellent ones available, we have highlighted the key concepts that should be addressed in each policy area.

Other topics your agency should consider developing into an SOP include the following:

- Use of emergency warning devices
- Parking and securing a vehicle
- Basic defensive driving
- Service animal transportation
- Nonemergency driving
- Emergency driving

- The regional traffic incident management system (TIMS)
- Education and training requirements for your service

## Backing of the EMS Vehicle

It is estimated that 25% of all emergency vehicle crashes occur while the emergency vehicle is operating in reverse. The average emergency vehicle operator may travel thousands of miles going forward. This same EVO will back up only 1 or 2 miles per year. The ratio of time or miles spent driving in reverse to the percentage of collisions is very concerning. We have a serious problem when we shift into reverse. Therefore, considerations in developing a backing policy should include the following:

- Backing should be avoided whenever possible. Where backing is unavoidable, a spotter, outside the vehicle, should be used even when backup cameras are present. Only emergency services personnel should be used to do this. If a patient is on board and a spotter is not outside, then the EMS member with the patient should get out and spot the vehicle, provided that they are not actively engaged in patient care.
- When placing the vehicle in reverse, the horn should be tapped twice to let your spotter and everyone else around know you are about to back up. In addition, the reverse alarm should be functional every time the vehicle is placed in reverse.
- If no qualified spotter is available, whenever possible, the EVO should park the vehicle, get out, and make a complete 360-degree survey of the space cushion around all four sides of the vehicle to locate any obstructions or hazards present before backing the emergency vehicle.
- Spotters are *never* permitted to ride the tailgates or running boards, or hang off the rear of any emergency vehicle in motion. Spotters should be located to the driver's side rear of the emergency vehicle in a safe position so they can be observed in the operator's mirror.
- Spotters should use the proper hand signals when the emergency vehicle is being backed. Uniform hand signals should be established as part of the backing policy. (Refer to Figure 4-15 for images of sample hand signals.)
- The emergency vehicle should not be backed until the spotter is in the proper safe position and communicates via voice or visible signal to the operator. The spotter should always be visible to the EVO in the safe zone. If the emergency vehicle operator loses sight of the spotter, the vehicle should

## CRASH ANALYSIS

### Ambulance Struck from Behind in Missouri

This crash was a multi-vehicle event involving a 2012 Freightliner M2 Type I ambulance and a 1999 Jeep Grand Cherokee that resulted in serious injuries to the ambulance's unbelted 27-year-old male paramedic, its 61-year-old male unbelted driver, and its 48-year-old male patient who was restrained to a cot. The weather was partly cloudy with a temperature of 86°F. The driver of the Jeep was a 60-year-old female who was unbelted. The Jeep and Freightliner were traveling north on a four-lane divided interstate highway when the front of the Jeep struck the left rear corner of the Freightliner ambulance. The speed limit was 70 mph and the ambulance was in the right lane traveling at 65 mph when it was struck by the Jeep. The impact redirected the ambulance off the road into a guard-rail end terminal and the front struck a median cable barrier. This caused the ambulance to roll onto its right side. The Jeep continued north on the highway and struck the east and west guardrails. The ambulance was transporting the patient without its emergency warning lights or siren in use at the time. Following the crash all three occupants of the ambulance and the Jeep's driver were transported by ambulances to hospitals. The Jeep driver's toxicology screening at the ED was positive for alcohol. The ambulance EVO sustained lumbar spine fractures, major scalp lacerations, closed head injury, and a clavicle fracture and was admitted to the hospital. The paramedic was flown by helicopter to the Level I trauma center and hospitalized for 24 days before transfer to a rehab center. The injuries he sustained included thoracic vertebral fractures with complete spinal cord injury, bilateral posterior-medial rib fractures, right hemopneumothorax, bilateral pulmonary contusions, a large posterior mediastinal hematoma, right clavicle fracture, displacement of the right acromioclavicular joint and soft tissue injuries of the back, shoulder and hip areas. The patient was being transported for a medical incident and had been fully immobilized and secured to the cot system. His medical records were not released to the investigator at the time of this report.

The municipal ambulance agency was a multitiered medical transport service. It was capable of providing all levels of EMS care. The agency covers a 181 square mile area of Missouri and performs public emergency response, interfacility transfers, and specialty transports using a fleet of 14 Type I ambulances. The agency requires its employees who operate vehicles to complete EVO training and the driver in this crash had taken the training many times as well as been an instructor for the in-house training. The service has a fatigue SOP that allows employees to take extended breaks for rest and/or leave work early at their request if the medical professional starts feeling fatigued.

1. How could this crash have been prevented?
2. Does your agency have an SOP for seat belt use of EVO?
3. Does your agency have an SOP for restraint of the patient and personnel in the patient compartment?

Modified from Crash Research & Analysis. *Special Crash Investigations: On-Site Ambulance Crash Investigation; Vehicle: 2012 Freightliner M2 Type I Ambulance; Location: Missouri; Crash Date: July 2020* (Report No. DOT HS 813 290). National Highway Traffic Safety Administration. May 2022. https://crashstats.nhtsa.dot.gov/Api/Public/ViewPublication/813290

be stopped immediately. When the spotter is in the proper/safe position, the emergency vehicle can continue to back up.

- Backing should be done very slowly and with great caution. The vehicle's speed should be controlled with the brake and not the accelerator.

There are some general rules for EVOs and spotters to always consider when backing the vehicle:

- Never be in a rush when backing or parking.
- Do not start to back or park when unsure of the area.
- Do not put the emergency vehicle into reverse gear until it has come to a complete stop.
- When it is dark, use the side and rear spotlights when backing.

- Backup alarms and/or backup cameras should be in the on position at all times, especially when backing the emergency vehicle.
- When turning while backing, check front fender swing to avoid front-end collisions.

Finally, all EVOs should practice backing the vehicle during their training. Start with backing between cones into a simulated garage. Try backing around the serpentine cone setup, and then practice backing into the garage at the EMS station. The only acceptable time for not using a spotter when backing is on the driving range when there is a safety officer assuring all personnel are in a safe zone away from the rear of the vehicles and the only thing that could be struck is a cone or two.

---

## Use of Seat belts and Restraints

As EMS practitioners, we know better than the general public the traumatic and often fatal effects of automobile crashes. The lifesaving impact of seat belts and restraints has been well researched and proven by National Highway Traffic Safety Administration (NHTSA). Most states have passed laws requiring drivers and the occupants of vehicles to be belted when the vehicle is in motion. Some states have included an emergency vehicle waiver in their seat belt law.

In regard to the front compartment of an ambulance, there is no acceptable reason for the EVO to waive the seat belt requirement. If a family member is allowed to ride along to the hospital, it should be the EVO's responsibility to make sure the person is properly belted. If the individual refuses to wear a seat belt, it is best to not allow them to ride in the ambulance, as the individual could be seriously injured if the ambulance should be involved in a collision.

### SAFETY TIP

To ensure that any friend or family member of the patient is safely restrained, the EVO should assist the individual in buckling up prior to driving to the hospital.

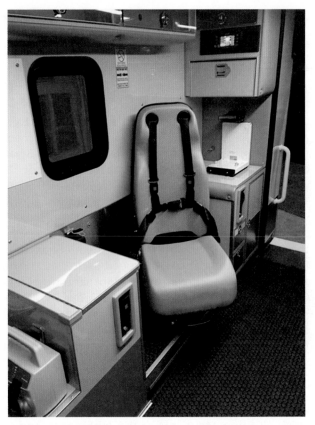

**Figure 12-2** Safety seat with full harness belting.
© Jones & Bartlett Learning. Courtesy of Bob Elling.

When there are EMS practitioners or any family members in the patient compartment of the ambulance and the vehicle is in motion, they should have their seat belt on. Even though it is often legal for the crew to be unrestrained in the patient compartment, it is *never* recommended. Some would argue that it is not always possible to be belted in when providing care to the patient. In reality, this is a very rare occurrence, and the manufacturers of ambulances are working on developing seats in tracks that can restrain the EMS practitioner while providing care (**Figure 12-2**).

Many EMS practitioners believe that the cargo net hanging at the end of the bench seat is a restraint device. There are some who even refer to it as the "medic catcher," since they believe it will hang intact and protect the practitioner from coming off the bench seat and hitting the cabinets that are normally across the doorway from the bench seat. Some practitioners also use the cargo net as a storage device, from which to hang cleaning sprays, quick-access packs, stethoscopes, and other items. Hanging objects from the cargo net makes it unsafe as a restraint device, and its ability to hold a practitioner in place during a collision is doubtful since, as some collision videos depict, the force of the practitioner's impact can cause the netting to come free. The

cargo net should neither be considered a restraint device nor used as a storage device as shown in **Figure 12-3**.

The patient should always be properly restrained in the seat belts on the stretcher, including the over-the-shoulder restraint (**Figure 12-4**). If a pediatric patient is transported in the ambulance, they should be restrained in a properly sized car seat or in appropriate strapping on the stretcher (**Figure 12-5**). Car seats are not made or rated to be placed in lateral positions, such as on the bench seat or in the CPR seat; they need to be on the cot or in the airway seat (at the head of the stretcher). With an integrated child restraint system, the airway seat opens into a child safety seat, which can be used to transport a child who is uninjured or who does not require continuous and/or intensive medical monitoring and/or interventions (**Figure 12-6**).

## Use of Emergency Lights at an Incident on a Roadway

Since many emergency lighting packages have different settings that can be used to maximize visibility in different ambient conditions, each department should have an SOP and provide training for EVOs in emergency lighting

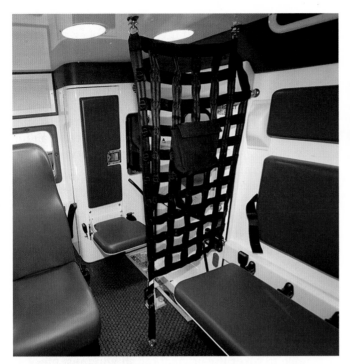

**Figure 12-3** The cargo net is not an effective restraint device.
Courtesy of Crestline Coach Ltd

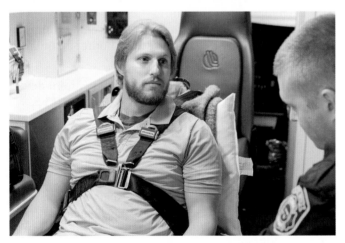

**Figure 12-4** A patient with shoulder straps properly applied.
© Jones & Bartlett Learning. Photographed by Darren Stahlman.

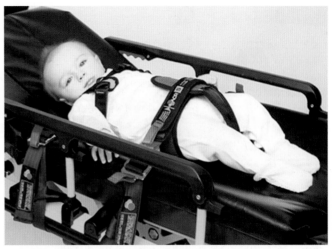

**Figure 12-5** An injured child should be transported in an appropriately sized child restraint system on the stretcher.
Courtesy of Evac+Chair International Ltd

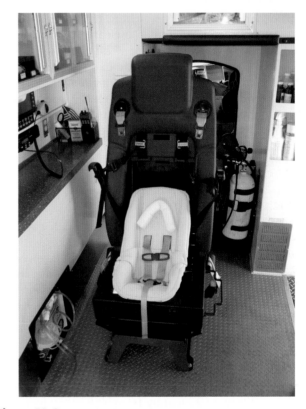

**Figure 12-6** An integrated child restraint system.
Courtesy of Serenity Safety Products

package capabilities and usage. Guidelines to include in an SOP include the following:

- Use emergency lights to provide warning and promote move-over behavior.
- Reduce forward-facing lights to mitigate opposite direction distractions and delays, as well as minimize potential blinding effects for oncoming motorists.
- Only display lights on vehicles blocking travel lanes and/or only on the rear-most vehicle when multiple response vehicles are on the shoulder.

## Safety on the Driving Range

When a skills course is set up to complement the didactic component of the EVOS course, it is imperative that this exercise be treated as a potentially dangerous event and that all care is taken when one or more vehicles are on

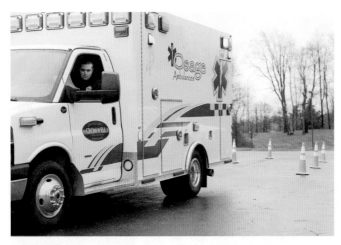

**Figure 12-7** An EMS practitioner backing the ambulance on the range into some cones.
© Jones & Bartlett Learning. Photographed by Darren Stahlman.

the driving range. Do not assume that any EVO, regardless of experience level, is watching the other students at the range. Exercises should be clearly explained and demonstrated by the driver trainer. The EVO should then be allowed to practice the specific exercise (e.g., backing into a cone garage, serpentine maneuvers forward and backward, parallel parking the vehicle) without any other students on the driving range. It is not necessary to practice with a spotter in the backing exercises as seen in **Figure 12-7**.

There should be a clearly marked safety zone for other students in the class to stay within while awaiting their turn. EVOs who are driving the vehicles should stay away from the safety zones.

The training area should be large enough and free of obstacles to allow students to make mistakes without any consequences and without placing themselves or others in danger. As a rule, the range should be a minimum of 10 times the vehicle's length, and the width of the maneuver should include the total turning radius and the safe zone. The safe zone should be calculated as turning radius (TR) $\times$ $\frac{2}{3}$ $\times$ 2. The purpose of multiplying by 2 is to account for each side of the maneuver. For example, if working with a vehicle that is 25 feet long, we would determine the minimum length of our field by multiplying 25 feet by 10, which is 250 feet. The proper minimum safe zone for a vehicle with a 30-foot turning radius would be calculated as 30 feet $\times$ .66 $\times$ 2, which is 40 feet (20 feet for each side of the maneuver). The total width of the training area would then be 70 feet (30 feet + 40 feet).

## Encountering a Collision

In the course of responding to a call, ambulances may encounter another collision along the way. There are several steps that should be taken to ensure that the best outcome is achieved for all involved. A policy should be developed, which includes the following steps:

1. Stop to investigate immediately, inform dispatch of the exact location and that you are assessing the situation and may be delayed to the original call. If first responders or police are on the scene, determine if you are needed or if they can wait for another ambulance and you can proceed to the original call.
2. If no police or first responders are on the scene, check patients for injuries.
3. Notify dispatch with location, number, type and extent of injuries, and any need for additional units and police.
4. Protect the incident scene with warning devices (e.g., cones) to prevent additional damage or injuries.
5. Do not move the vehicles until the police have arrived.
6. If collision involves non–life-threatening injuries, check with dispatcher to see if another unit is available to cover the original call. If you must proceed to the original call wait until the first responding unit arrives and inform them they need to wait for another ambulance to arrive as you must proceed to a higher priority call.
7. If life-threatening injuries are present, administer aid and notify dispatch to send another ambulance to the original call.

## Procedures Following a Crash

Unfortunately, at some point, each service will experience an ambulance collision (**Figure 12-8**). An emergency vehicle collision can present a major problem for an agency, but that problem can be greatly intensified if practitioners do not know how to regain control of the situation or are not aware of any plans to deal with a collision. An SOP for responding to crashes should include the following steps:

1. Notify the dispatcher right away and have the police, your supervisor, and other emergency services respond as necessary.
2. Determine whether there are injuries and whether an ambulance will be needed at the scene to treat and transport the injured, including your patient if you are carrying one.
3. Notify the dispatcher if the call you were responding to will require another unit to be sent in your place.
4. In most cases, it makes the most sense not to move the vehicles until the police have had the opportunity to document the scene. Moving the vehicles could have a detrimental effect on the

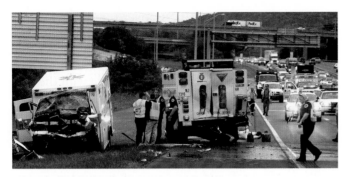

**Figure 12-8** An ambulance crash scene.
© Larry McCormack/The Tennessean/AP Photo

investigation. Some states may have laws requiring vehicles to be moved out of traffic and not impede the traffic if there were no injuries involved; the SOP must follow state and local laws. If vehicles must be moved, take photos of the scene (not the damage) from a relative distance; try to include any road signs or markings and any geographic factors (e.g., hills, curves) that may have contributed to the collision. Also, mark the roadway at each point of the tires using the "T" method of a line alongside the tire and a line protruding out from the center hub. This helps in identifying the vehicles' positions.

5.  Assign someone to deal with traffic appropriately until the police can take over that duty. Set up the proper flare or cone configuration that will assist motorists in identifying the collision and clearly move them away from the immediate area. Do not use flares when there are gasoline or other flammable liquid spills.

6.  If the ambulance will need to be towed to a garage or body shop, make sure the drug box, HIPAA-protected documentation, and expensive equipment are removed and secured.

7.  Services should have a policy that no personnel, except a designated public information officer, may talk to the media. Statements made while under duress could be inappropriate and come back at you or your service in a negative way.

8.  If there is any injury, regardless of how minor, it should be evaluated at the time of the collision and not left until the following day. A worker's compensation package should be completed no matter how minuscule the injury.

9.  All pertinent insurance information should be gathered as it would if the collision happened in a personal vehicle.

10. If law enforcement or department policies require a breathalyzer or field sobriety tests, make sure they are done out of the view of the public and news teams. Many times, these are standard practices that can reflect poorly on the agency if shown in the media.

## Visibility at the Scene

Traffic is a serious threat to the health and safety of the EMS practitioners and the EVO when working at the scene on a roadway. Whenever possible, law enforcement personnel will take responsibility for rerouting, stopping, or diverting traffic away from the EMS personnel and patients. All personnel must wear highly visible apparel, provided by the agency/department, when working in traffic on the roadway. As discussed previously, use of emergency lights on scene should also be outlined.

## Qualifications for New Emergency Vehicle Operators

Your agency/department should clearly spell out what type of individual it is looking for as an applicant to become trained as an EVO. Considerations should include minimum age, years driving and clean record, maturity and good sense of responsibility, physical fitness, and dedication to improving driving skills.

The minimum duration and the specific objectives of the training program should be clearly spelled out. All EVO candidates need to understand the commitment they are making to become qualified.

It should be written in the SOP that the service will be conducting background checks of employees'/members' driver's licenses at the time of their initial application and/or qualification as an EVO as well as on a regular basis. It is the responsibility of the EVO to make the leadership of the agency aware of any serious infractions (points, moving violations, suspensions, crashes with injuries, DWIs/DWAIs) that occur while not at work at the agency. Many departments and states will require vehicle operators to carry their own automobile insurance even though they are covered by the department while working.

## No Distractions While Driving Policy

Most states have already passed laws prohibiting talking on a cell phone and texting while driving because they take the driver's attention and hands away from vehicle operation. Yet, it is common to drive down the highway and notice an EVO talking on a cell phone, talking on the radio, or in some instances texting or operating the computer in the front of the ambulance. These are all distractions and can lead to a very serious crash. If you must use the phone, pull the vehicle over to a safe spot to use your cell phone to check in with your family or friends or dispatch; do not do so while you are cruising down the highway.

As much as possible, eliminating the distractions to the EVO will help improve the safety of the ride to and from the call. Some services make it the responsibility of the crew member in the cab, who is not the driver, to deal with the radio transmissions and the maps or GPS devices while en route to the scene. Other distractions you may want to consider include eating, drinking, and grooming while driving.

The bottom line is that your SOP should be written in such a way as to minimize the distraction and create a sterile cab for the emergency vehicle operator.

## Zero Tolerance for Alcohol and Drugs

The majority of EMS and fire service agencies employ a **zero tolerance** approach to substance use, strictly prohibiting any members or employees from responding to a call, or participating in any operational or support aspect of the organization, while under the influence of alcohol. According to the International Association of Fire Chiefs' (IAFC) policy statement, Drug and Alcohol-Free Awareness (2012), "No member of a fire and emergency services agency/organization shall participate in any operational or support aspect of the organization while under the influence of alcohol, including but not limited to, any fire and emergency operations, fire-police, training, administrative functions, rehab, etc." The statement recommends that agencies develop written policies and have procedures in place for testing the blood alcohol levels of any individual involved in an incident that results in "measurable damage to apparatus or property; or injury/death of civilians or agency/organization personnel." The IAFC also suggests that members not consume alcohol within 8 hours of performing any emergency services duties, and if they are still impaired by alcohol consumed more than 8 hours previously, they should voluntarily remove themselves from service until they have fully recovered. It additionally recommends that agencies obtain legal advice and create policies that take into account the use of social halls for both department and nondepartment functions.

Prescription and illicit drugs are also included in the IAFC's recommendations. Its position is that drug abuse should not be tolerated regardless of the type of drug, that there should also be zero tolerance of illegal drugs, and that agencies should have policies in place to test and suspend personnel during internal or external investigations. Prescription or over-the-counter drugs used while on duty should be approved by a healthcare professional and reported to a supervisor, who should verify that over-the-counter medications are allowed by the department physician and the safe use with the prescribing physician in the case of prescription drugs. The IAFC also suggests that Employee Assistance Programs be made available to members who are dealing with drug and alcohol abuse.

With the increasing number of states that have legalized medical and recreational marijuana usage, SOPs should be updated to reflect agency policy on off-duty use. Laws and regulations vary widely from state to state, so legal counsel should be involved to ensure that SOPs are in compliance with all regulations, especially those regarding disability-related protections and any statutes specific to EMS or other safety-sensitive workplaces.

Each service's medical director, leadership and representatives from human resources, safety and risk department, and employee association or union should come to an agreement on a reasonable policy in reference to drugs, including prescription and over-the-counter medications, which can impair the EVO's driving abilities.

## Reporting Work-Related Injuries, Illnesses, and Near Misses

Every agency must have a clear SOP that spells out the procedure for reporting all work-related injuries/illnesses, no matter the severity. Occupational Safety and Health Administration (OSHA) legislation requires employers to keep records of certain injuries and illnesses, and to report certain workplace incidents to OSHA within specific time periods.

Aside from these worker's compensation–related reports, there are often incidents that could have been serious but did not trigger a reporting requirement. Such "near misses" can serve as lessons that can be learned to help prevent future actual incidents should these incidents be properly and confidentially shared. Each agency should have an SOP on reporting near misses, be it to supervision and/or to a national database. The policy should address roles and responsibilities, as well as a statement on nonretaliation toward the member/employee involved in the incident. **Appendix 12-B** provides a template for a near-miss SOP. See Chapter 8, *Crash Prevention*, for more information on near misses and reporting systems.

## SUMMARY

- EVOs must understand how and why agencies develop SOPs.
- Emergency services should develop a clear policy for backing the emergency vehicle.
- Emergency services should clearly define requirements for the use of seat belts and restraints in the emergency vehicle.
- Safety precautions must be in place whenever driving skills are being practiced at the driving range.
- Emergency services should clearly state the specifics that EVOs should follow if involved in a collision while operating the emergency vehicle or encountering a collision while on the road.
- A department policy should exist in regard to visibility on the scene of an emergency call and lighting at the incident.

- Emergency services should clearly define the requirements for practitioners to become qualified as EVOs.
- A clear policy should be in place for eliminating distractions to the EVO while operating an emergency vehicle.
- All EMS agencies must have a zero-tolerance policy in place for substances that affect EVOs' coordination and judgment when operating an emergency vehicle.
- All employees should be aware of the policy on reporting injuries/illness and near misses while at work.

## GLOSSARY

**SMART objectives** An acronym that describes the key characteristics of meaningful objectives: *s*pecific, *m*easurable, *a*chievable, *r*ealistic, and *t*ime-bound.

**standard operating procedure (SOP)** A policy issued by an agency's leadership to spell out how the employees or members are expected to perform in a specific instance or circumstance.

**zero tolerance** A policy that makes a given behavior absolutely unacceptable; unlike a "three strikes" rule, only one infraction is necessary to trigger disciplinary actions.

## RESOURCES

Center for Patient Safety. EVENT: An EMS Voluntary Notification Tool from EMSForward. Retrieved from https://www.emsforward.org/event

Cumberland Valley Volunteer Fireman's Association & Emergency Responder Safety Institute. (2018). *Study of protecting emergency responders on the highways and operation of emergency vehicles: A review of first responder agencies who have adopted emergency lighting and vehicle conspicuity technology.* Retrieved from https://www.respondersafety.com/Download.aspx?id=fa2f464f-2498-4741-917b-809592fcd789

Department of Homeland Security, Science and Technology Directorate, First Responders Group. (2013). *A research study of ambulance operations and best practice considerations for emergency medical services personnel.* Retrieved from https://www.dhs.gov/sites/default/files/publications/Ambulance%20Driver%20%28Operator%29%20Best%20Practices%20Report.pdf

McNeil and Company, Ambulance Driving Policy Guidelines. Retrieved from https://www.mcneilandcompany.com/risk-management/resources/

National Fire Fighter Near-Miss Reporting System. www.firefighternearmiss.com

U.S. Department of Transportation, National Highway Traffic Safety Administration. (2012). Working group best-practice recommendations for the safe transportation of children in emergency ground ambulances. DOT HS 811 677. Retrieved from https://preventinjury.pediatrics.iu.edu/wp-content/uploads/2023/03/Article-NHTSA-Best-Practices-Safe-Transport-Children-201209.pdf

# REFERENCES

Crash Research & Analysis, Inc. (2022, May). *Special Crash Investigations: On-site ambulance crash investigation; Vehicle: 2012 Freightliner M2 Type I Ambulance; Location: Missouri; Crash Date: July 2020* (Report No. DOT HS 813 290). NHTSA. Retrieved from https://crashstats.nhtsa.dot.gov/Api/Public/ViewPublication/813290

Federal Emergency Management Agency & U.S. Fire Administration. (1999). Developing Effective Standard Operating Procedures For Fire and EMS Departments (FA-197/December 1999). Retrieved from https://www.in.gov/dhs/files/effectivesop.pdf

International Association of Fire Chiefs. (n.d.). Template: Near-miss reporting SOP. Retrieved from https://www.iafc.org/topics-and-tools/resources/resource/template-near-miss-reporting-sop

International Association of Fire Chiefs. (2012). Position statement: drug and alcohol-free awareness. Retrieved from https://www.iafc.org/topics-and-tools/resources/resource/iafc-position-drug-and-alcohol-free-awareness

Occupational Safety and Health Administration. (2021). Near miss reporting policy. Retrieved from https://www.osha.gov/sites/default/files/2021-07/Template%20for%20Near%20Miss%20Reporting%20Policy.pdf

Rukavina, J. "Shrooms and smoke signals": Legal drugs in the firehouse. *FireRescue1*. Retrieved from https://www.firerescue1.com/legal/articles/shrooms-and-smoke-signals-legal-drugs-in-the-firehouse-kybxZ7UF1RtVnPdA/

# Appendix 12-A Overview of SOP Topic Areas

## Management and Administration

### General Administration

- Organization
- Facilities
- Emergency Vehicles and Specialized Apparatus
- Equipment and Supplies
- Finance
- Fundraising
- Training, Education, and Exercises
- Information Management

### Member Health and Assistance Programs

- Medical Screening/Health Assessment
- Health and Wellness Promotion
- Performance Evaluation
- Post-Injury Rehabilitation
- Employee/Member Assistance
- Facility Safety
- Hazard Communication

### Organizational Planning and Preparedness

- Strategic/Master Planning
- SOP Development
- Risk Management
- Emergency Operations Planning
- Mutual/Automatic Aid

## Prevention and Special Programs

### Public Information and Education

- Working with the Public
- Working with the Media
- Emergency Public Information
- Public Education
- Public Relations

## Building Inspections and Codes Enforcement

- Authorities and Codes
- Design and Plans Review
- Residential Inspections
- Commercial Inspections
- Industrial Inspections
- Code Enforcement
- Record Keeping

### Special Programs

- Fire Cause and Arson Investigation
- Hydrant Maintenance
- Other Special Programs

## Emergency Operations

### General Emergency Operations

- Operating Emergency Vehicles
- Safety at Emergency Incidents
- Communications
- Command and Control
- Special Operations
- Post-Incident Operations

### Fire Suppression

- Fire Suppression Risk Management
- Company Operations
- Tactical/Strategic Guidelines
- Special Facilities/Target Hazards
- Special Fire Suppression Operations

### Emergency Medical Response

- EMS Response Risk Management
- Pre-hospital EMS First Response
- Patient Disposition and Transportation
- Management of EMS Operations
- Special EMS Operations

## Hazardous Materials Response

- Hazmat Response Risk Management
- First Responder Operations
- Special Hazmat Operations

## Technical Rescue

- Technical Rescue Risk Management
- Rescue Operations
- Special Rescue Operations

## Disaster Operations

- Organizing for Disaster Operations
- Disaster Operations Risk Management
- Disaster Operations
- Disaster-Specific Guidelines

# Appendix 12-B Model SOP for Near-Miss Reporting

| Your Department / Agency Logo | Your Department / Agency Name | | |
|---|---|---|---|
| | **Policy #** | **Effective Date** | Chief's Signature |
| | **Subject:** Near-Miss Reporting * | | |

## Background

Near-miss reporting has proven to reduce fatalities, injuries, and equipment loss in a number of industries (i.e., aviation, medicine, gas/oil, nuclear). Managing error through the use of nonpunitive strategies such as near-miss reporting has proven to be an effective tool in keeping the workforce and community served safe. Given the concept's proven track record and the dedication this department/ agency has to the health and welfare of its members/ employees, the (your department/agency name here) is issuing this policy endorsing the use of near-miss reporting.

## Applicability

This policy applies to all members/employees of the (your department/agency name).
*An endorsement from the jurisdiction's labor group or governing body should be placed here.*

## Definitions

- E.V.E.N.T.—The (EMS Voluntary Event Notification Tool) is a tool designed to improve the safety, quality, and consistent delivery of emergency medical services. It collects data submitted anonymously by EMS practitioners.
- Near-miss event—A near-miss event is defined as an unintentional unsafe occurrence that could have resulted in an injury, fatality, or property damage. Only a fortunate break in the chain of events prevented an injury, fatality, or damage.
- Near-Miss Reporting System—The National Fire Fighter Near-Miss Reporting System (www .firefighternearmiss.com) is a voluntary, confidential, nonpunitive, and secure reporting system with the goal of improving firefighter/EMT safety. By collecting and analyzing information on near-miss events, improvements can be made in command, education, operations, and training.

- Reporter—Someone who files a near-miss report.
- Reviewer—A contract employee of www .firefighternearmiss.com hired to review near-miss reports and collect data. Reviewers sign confidentiality agreements as a condition of employment by the National Fire Fighter Near-Miss Reporting System. Reviewers are active or recently retired fire service members with at least 15 years of experience.

## Policy

The (your department/agency name) is adopting a nonpunitive approach to human error. Members/employees who commit an error while in the performance of their duty shall be exempt from disciplinary action provided they promptly file a near-miss report. This exemption from disciplinary action applies to actions that do not willfully violate department/agency SOP or purposely place members/employees or citizens unnecessarily in harm's way.

Members/employees who personally experience, witness, or are made aware of a near-miss event shall file a near-miss report.

Members/employees filing near-miss reports shall use either the National Fire Fighter Near-Miss Reporting System (www.firefighternearmiss.com) or the EVENT system (https://event.clirems.org/Near-Miss-Event) as the vehicle for recording their near-miss event.

Multiple reports of the same incident are encouraged. The variety of perspectives provides additional value to reporting the incident.

Members/employees are encouraged to forward a copy of the posted report to the Department/Agency Safety Office so the department/agency can rapidly respond to implement corrective actions needed to prevent the near miss from becoming a serious injury or fatality within our department/agency.

Ensuring anonymity and confidentiality is paramount. No member/employee submitting a near-miss report shall be forced to identify themselves. Department/

agency management shall not seek out the identity of a member(s)/employee(s) who file near-miss reports. Members/employees who voluntarily submit their contact information to the department/agency will remain anonymous.

## Procedure

Members/employees who experience, witness, or are informed of a near-miss incident shall submit the report to www.firefighternearmiss.com or the EVENT system (https://www.emsforward.org/event) to support the program's efforts to improve EMS practitioner safety.

Sections 1 thru 4 of www.firefighternearmiss.com or the EVENT system form at https://www.emsforward.org/event shall be completed by the affected/informed members/employees.

Section 5 of the reporting system is optional. Members/employees are *encouraged* to provide at least one off-duty contact number or email address. This contact information provides the system's reviewers with a means to contact the reporter with follow-up questions that will enhance the data collected and provide the maximum reporting effort to ensure another practitioner's safety.

Reporters may copy their submitted report and send it to the department/agency safety officer or they may wait until the report is posted. No names or contact information are required at the department/agency level.

## Responsibility

Management is responsible for ensuring the department/agency maintains a non-punitive approach to correcting errors.

Department/agency officers are responsible for maintaining an environment that encourages members/employees to report errors and file near-miss reports.

All members/employees are responsible for filing timely near-miss reports.

All officers are responsible for maintaining a working knowledge of the National Fire Fighter Near-Miss Reporting System or the EVENT system (depending which is used by this department/agency).

The department/agency safety officer is responsible for filing reports with www.firefighternearmiss.com or EVENT system (https://event.clirems.org/Near-Miss-Event) whenever they are notified or becomes aware of a near-miss event in the department/agency.

**\* NOTE:**
This sample SOP is based on the model policy provided by the National Fire Fighter Near-Miss Reporting System. It refers to both the firefighter near-miss system as well as the EVENT system provided by the Center for Leadership, Innovation and Research in EMS (CLIR) in partnership with NAEMT, NASEMSO, and the National EMS Management Association. When deciding to adapt this model SOP each department/agency should select the most appropriate reporting system to use.

Modified from International Association of Fire Chiefs. Template: near-miss reporting SOP. May 1, 2012. https://www.iafc.org/topics-and-tools/resources/resource/template-near-miss-reporting-sop

# Glossary

**4-5-12 rule** A recommendation to maintain a 4-second interval between your vehicle and the vehicle ahead for speeds below 55 mph, increasing the following distance to 5 seconds for traveling speeds above 55 mph, and encompassing a 12-second visual lead time.

**active training** The portion of training in which a student develops the answers through facilitated learning instead of instruction.

**advanced warning area** Area established to warn motorists of an approaching incident and allow them to prepare for the new traffic control pattern.

**air brakes** A braking system that uses air as a medium for applying the brakes.

**air horn** A warning device that uses compressed air, which is either electronically or manually controlled, to emit a unidirectional, long-range, low-frequency warning sound.

**alternators** Electromechanical devices that convert mechanical energy to electrical energy in the form of alternating current; automotive alternators use a set of rectifiers mechanical energy to electrical energy in the form of alternating current; automotive alternators use a set of rectifiers to convert alternating current to direct current to charge the vehicle batteries.

**Ambulance Accident Prevention Seminar (AAPS)** A course launched in 1989 by the New York State Department of Health to help improve attitudes toward emergency vehicle operation.

**antilock brakes** A computerized braking system that prevents wheel lockup, helping the vehicle maintain directional control.

**batteries** Devices that chemically store electrical energy; they are generally used for starting the vehicle and short-term electrical use.

**black box** A monitoring recorder, found on commercial aircraft, also called a flight recorder. Similar types of electronic devices are often found in emergency vehicles to provide a recording of events leading up to the moments when a crash occurred.

**black ice** A thin film of water frozen on the road.

**blind spots** Areas that prevent the driver from seeing the path or presence of an object.

**block** To position a fire department apparatus on an angle to the lanes of traffic, creating a physical barrier between upstream traffic and the work area. Includes block to the left and block to the right.

**brake fade** A condition in which brakes become ineffective secondary to heat buildup in the braking system.

**braking distance** The physical stopping distance of the vehicle once the brakes are applied.

**braking system** The entire system that allows the vehicle operator to stop the vehicle by applying pressure to the vehicle's brake pedal.

**buffer space** The area immediately after the transition area, in which the traffic begins to slow down and move out of the incident lane.

**camber** The banking of the roadway; an arched road surface.

**Centers for Disease Control and Prevention (CDC)** The government agency that works to protect American health, safety, and security from all types of diseases, including those caused by human error and preventable problems.

**chevron** An inverted V-shaped striping that slants downward at a 45-degree angle and reflects light; it is applied to the rear of emergency vehicles to increase visibility.

**civil law** The type of law that pertains to determining responsibility for a wrongful act and imposing monetary penalties (with or without criminal charges) if the defendant is found guilty.

**Coaching the Emergency Vehicle Operator (CEVO)** An emergency vehicle operation course offered by the National Safety Council; it launched in the early 1990s and was updated to CEVO-4 in 2021.

**conspicuity** The quality of being clearly discernable and easy to see.

**contour** The curvature of a roadway.

**criminal law** The type of law that pertains to determining whether a statute has been violated and, if so, imposing a punishment (fine and/or imprisonment) on the guilty party.

**crown** The slope of a roadway, designed to facilitate drainage of water and debris.

**defendant** The person or party in a lawsuit who is charged with breaking the law and harming the plaintiff.

**disc brakes** A braking system designed with a disc and a brake caliper installed over the disc.

**downstream** In regard to the direction of travel, the area after the incident, where traffic is moving away from the incident.

**driver behavior monitoring systems (DBMSs)** See *driver monitoring devices.*

**driver monitoring devices** Monitoring systems that track driver actions, vehicle movement, and immediate environment around the vehicle using video cameras and sensors.

**driving simulator** A training tool used in driver's education courses to expose students to realistic driving situations and to assess driver behavior and human factors. Typically, simulators involve a computer display of everything the operator would see through the windshield and mirrors during actual driving.

**drum brakes** A braking system that has a circular wheel hub with two semicircular brake shoes installed inside.

**due regard** Appropriate consideration and responsibility shown for the safety of others.

**electrical system** The system that generates and maintains electrical energy required for vehicle operation as well as for patient care activities.

**electronic stability control (ESC)** Computerized system used to detect and mitigate skids. When an ESC system identifies a loss of steering control, it automatically applies the brakes, and may cut engine power, to help control and direct the vehicle.

**Emergency Vehicle Driving Training (EVDT)** An emergency vehicle operation course offered by the Volunteer Fireman's Insurance Services (VFIS); it was launched in 1980 and updated in 2016.

**Emergency Vehicle Operator Course (EVOC)** A course launched in 1978 by the U.S. Department of Transportation to reduce the incidence of emergency vehicle collisions.

**emergency vehicle operator (EVO)** The individual driving the emergency vehicle, generally an ambulance, who has the ability to operate it in the emergency mode (activating the lights and/or siren).

**EMS Vehicle Operator Safety (EVOS)** A course launched in 1989 and updated in 2023, endorsed by the NAEMT, that is designed to promote a culture of safety, prepare EVOs, and reduce the risk of driving an emergency vehicle.

**engine** A device that provides the mechanical motive force for propelling a vehicle and powering its subsystems.

**evidence-based guidelines (EBGs)** Recommendations derived from the research to help define best practices and optimize decision making.

**exhaust system** The system for removing dangerous exhaust gases from the engine.

**fatigue** Refers to subjective physical and psychological symptoms that range from tiredness to exhaustion and interfere with a person's ability to function normally.

**Federal Q** A well-known and distinctive type of wail siren that is trademarked by Federal Signal Corporation.

**following distance** The distance between a vehicle and the vehicle ahead of it.

**friction** Resistance of an object to slide over another.

**geographic information system (GIS)** A computer system that combines database management system functionality with location information.

**georeferencing** The process of determining the location of data in physical space.

**global positioning system (GPS)** Satellite-based location and navigation system used to locate vehicles and provide directions to specific locations.

**gravity** A force that pulls objects toward the earth, resulting in what we know as weight.

**gross negligence** A more serious form of negligence that implies reckless conduct and a blatant disregard for the safety and lives of others. The line between negligence and gross negligence may need to be determined by a court.

**gross vehicle weight rating (GVWR)** The maximum allowable weight limit of a vehicle.

**high–low frequency siren** A siren sound with a sharp, clipped beginning and ending that cycles through higher and lower frequencies.

**hydraulic brakes** A braking system that uses fluid to charge and activate the brakes.

**hydroplaning** A driving situation in which a rolling tire rides up on a thin layer of water, preventing the tire tread from reaching the road surface.

**inertia** The resistance of an object to a change in its direction or speed.

**intersection marker light** The flashing emergency light on the side of the front fender, set at a 30-degree angle, that notifies motorists coming from a perpendicular direction in an intersection.

**inverters** Electrical devices that convert direct current to alternating current; they provide 110-volt current.

**kinetic energy** The energy of a moving object based on weight and speed.

**liability** Legal accountability or obligation.

**lights and siren (L&S)** The use of lights and siren sounds per policy of the agency in a presumed emergency response to the scene or transport destination.

**linear** Positioning a vehicle within or parallel to a lane of travel or shoulder to protect the incident scene. This providers a barrier only in the lane or shoulder in which the vehicle is parked and does little to funnel traffic; should be used in conjunction with block positioning.

**low-frequency siren** A proprietary siren that works in conjunction with the vehicle's existing siren by producing an extremely low frequency that can shake (rumble) nearby objects.

**maneuvering safety zone** An area where the vehicle operator can make mistakes and attempts at correcting them without the fear of hitting an obstacle.

**microsleeping** A brief break with consciousness in which a person loses awareness of their surroundings and momentarily enters a state of sleep.

**mobile data terminal (MDT)** A computerized device similar to a laptop computer that is used to communicate with a central dispatch office.

**morbidity** Illness or harm; a diseased state.

**mortality** Death; the quality of being mortal.

**MOST** Mnemonic that stands for *mirror, over (the shoulder), signal,* and *turn.* Used to remember the steps for safely changing lanes.

**moving left of center** A traffic law exemption in which the emergency vehicle crosses over a dividing line and travels in opposing traffic lanes.

**National Fire Protection Association (NFPA)** A standards-setting entity that develops gold standards for the fire service.

**National Highway Traffic Safety Administration (NHTSA)** An agency of the U.S. Department of Transportation responsible for ensuring safe driving conditions.

**near-miss program** A system that identifies situations that could have resulted in a collision in an effort to identify necessary revisions in procedures.

**near-miss recovery** The effectiveness with which the EVO recovers control of the ambulance after a near miss.

**negligence** Failure to exercise due caution.

**off-tracking** The offsetting of the rear wheels of the vehicle from the front wheels, as when the vehicle is turning.

**omnidirectional** A sound that travels in more than one direction and can cause confusion in identifying the location of the source.

**participant safety zone(s)** Safe locations within the proving ground that keep waiting participants out of the vehicle's trajectory and maneuvers.

**passive training** The portion of training in which a student receives instruction and is expected to glean knowledge from it rather than develop the knowledge on their own.

**payload** The total weight that a vehicle can carry within its gross vehicle weight rating.

**perception distance** The distance the vehicle travels while the driver perceives a change in traffic conditions.

**phaser** A proprietary siren with a unique ray gun sound.

**plaintiff** The person or party who files a complaint in a lawsuit claiming to have been harmed by the defendant.

**potential energy** The energy an object possesses while at rest.

**preponderance of the evidence** A requirement in determining the guilt of a defendant that the majority of evidence presented in a case favor the plaintiff's argument.

**preventable collision** A collision in which the driver failed to do everything reasonable to prevent its occurrence.

**preventive maintenance** Scheduled servicing, inspection, or replacement of specific items in the vehicle to reduce potential problems.

**reaction distance** The distance a vehicle travels during reaction time after perceiving a hazard but before applying the brakes.

**reasonable doubt** The lack of certainty that a person may justifiably feel based on the evidence at hand regarding the alleged guilt of a defendant.

**recognition-primed decision making (RPDM)** A process for how people can quickly make effective decisions in complex situations; based on using prior experiences to predict possible outcomes.

**recognize, process, and react** The process taken by motorists when acknowledging the presence of L&S; recognizing something out of the ordinary in the traffic environment, processing the change in traffic patterns and conditions, reacting by taking the appropriate action to avoid the collision/hazard identified.

**road rage** Aggressive or angry behavior by a driver of a motor vehicle that may include rude gestures, verbal insults or threats, or unsafe driving.

**roundabout** An intersection with a circular configuration that safely and efficiently moves traffic.

**safety cushion** An adequate vehicle clearance around all sides of the vehicle.

**safety officer** An assigned instructor to oversee all aspects of the range maneuvers and the safety of the instructors and students.

**sipes** Small slits in the tire tread that allow water to seep up within the tread block.

**sleep deprivation** The state of having an insufficient amount of sleep.

**SMART objectives** An acronym that describes the key characteristics of meaningful objectives: specific, measurable, achievable, realistic, and time-bound.

**standard operating procedure (SOP)** A policy issued by an agency's leadership to spell out how the employees or members are expected to perform in a specific instance or circumstance.

**"sterile" cockpit** A concept adapted from the airline industry in which, during critical phases of an operation, personnel are permitted to discuss only issues directly related to the task being performed. This approach increases awareness and decreases errors caused by inattention due to distraction.

**suspension system** The system that supports the vehicle and allows it to absorb the impact from bumpy roads without affecting the ride inside the cab and patient compartment.

**switchback maneuver** A series of sweeping left and right turns that allows the student to develop left- and right-side judgment and front-end depth perception.

**taper** To direct traffic to merge into adjacent lanes for the purposes of reducing the number of active travel lanes.

**temporary traffic control zone** An area of a roadway where normal traffic patterns have been temporarily changed; this can be due to an emergency incident, construction, special events, or maintenance of nearby structures (telephone lines, streetlights, etc.).

**traffic preemption systems** Systems used to preempt traffic lights, giving emergency vehicles the right-of-way.

**transition area** The space after the advanced warning area in which the traffic changes are implemented; warning devices are placed to direct motorists out of the incident lane(s) and into the new lanes of travel. Also known as the transition zone.

**transmission** A device that provides speed and torque conversions from the engine to the wheels using gear ratios; it reduces the higher engine speed to the slower wheel speed, increasing torque in the process.

**true emergency** A situation in which there is a high probability of death or serious injury to an individual or of significant property loss.

**turning radius** The width of the circle required for a vehicle to turn around without backing up.

**unidirectional** A sound that travels in one direction, aiding in identifying the location of the source.

**upstream** In regard to the direction of travel, the area before the incident, where traffic is moving toward the incident.

**valve stem** An opening to the valve that admits air to a tire and automatically closes to seal in pressure

**vehicle length** The total bumper-to-bumper length of the vehicle.

**virtual reality** A computer-based simulated environment through which users can interact with one another and their environment.

**wail** An undulating siren sound that is effective in notifying other motorists of your presence.

**wheelbase** The distance from the rear wheel hub to the front wheel hub.

**wheel track** The distance from the middle of the tread of one front tire to the middle of the tread of the other front tire.

**yelp** A siren sound that rises in pitch and has a short clip at the end, extremely effective for clearing intersections.

**zero tolerance** A policy that makes a given behavior absolutely unacceptable; unlike a "three strikes" rule, only one infraction is necessary to trigger disciplinary actions.

# Index

**Note:** Page numbers followed by "*b*", "*f*" and "*t*" refer to boxes, figure, and table respectively.